"In sharing her personal 'adventure' with cancer, as she so fittingly names it, Jackie Fox manages to educate and entertain her readers in a unique style that resonates with humor, gratitude and honesty. She has given voice to the numerous women who get thrown into a world of mixed messages and confusion following a diagnosis of DCIS-stage 0 cancer. As Jackie states, 'No one should tell us how to feel about our diagnosis,' and she reinforces this belief of individual choice throughout her story, reminding women to find their own path to peace."

—*Kathryn S. Gurland, LCSW, director/founder of PEG'S Group, LLC, Cancer Navigation Consultants who provide personal education, guidance and support for individuals affected by cancer, based in NYC*

"Jackie Fox has done an incredible job detailing her experience with stage 0 breast cancer. She's explained her journey, physical and emotional, in terms that everyone can understand and has provided invaluable tips for understanding the diagnosis and creating a treatment plan. '*From Zero to Mastectomy*' is a must-read for anyone recently diagnosed with stage 0 cancer."

—*Vicki Tashman, founder, Pink-Link, Connecting Breast Cancer Survivors Online*

From ZERO to Mastectomy:

What I Learned and You Need to Know About Stage 0 Breast Cancer

By Jackie Fox

Cover design: Janie Harting
Interior Design: WingSpan Press
Author photo: Scott Dobry Pictures
Editing: Katie Sosnowchik

Honyocker Press
P.O. Box 262
Gretna, Nebraska 68028
www.honyockerpress.com

Publisher's Cataloging-in-Publication Data

Fox, Jacqueline.
    From zero to mastectomy : what I learned and you need to know about stage 0 breast cancer / Jackie Fox.
        p. cm.
    ISBN: 978-0-578-05416-2
    1. Breast—Cancer—Patients—United States—Biography.
    2. Mastectomy—Patients—Biography.   I. Title.
RC280.B8 F69 2010
362.196`994490092—dc22

                                                        2010926806

For Bruce

I would maintain that thanks are the highest form of thought, and that gratitude is happiness doubled by wonder.

—*G.K. Chesterton*

Preface

If you're reading this, it's likely because stage 0 breast cancer has decided to show up in your life or the life of someone you love. If you're like I was, you don't have a clue what that means.

On the surface, getting stage 0 cancer is great news. It's not life-threatening if treated. But deciding on treatment is the tricky part; at least it was for me. When you're diagnosed with stage 3 or stage 4 cancer, there's no question you've got a fight on your hands. With stage 0, you may wonder, like I did, why some of the choices seem so drastic for a cancer that by definition is not invasive. You may wonder if you really are part of this club no one wants to join, and if you're entitled to call yourself a survivor. (Yes, and yes.)

I wrote this book because I want you to know you're not alone. Stage 0 breast cancer is very different from stage 2 or 3 or 4, yet some aspects of the cancer journey are universal. You're going to have days that suck, but those days don't have to define your experience. I remember feeling inexplicably happy one day while I was driving to work in the middle of my cancer adventure, and I couldn't come up with a reason—except maybe that it was good to be alive and driving to work. The birds were chirping and the sun was shining and I suddenly felt like a character in a Disney movie. I realized it doesn't take much more than that for life to be good. For you, the realization may hit while you're making cookies with your daughter or walking your dog. The simple moments can come to feel like blessings.

That's one thing I hope you take away from this book. The other thing is for you to be comfortable with the choices you make. Your doctors, treatment choices and favored coping strategies may not be anything like mine. Don't think you have to pattern your experience after mine or anyone else's. I did what worked for me and have no regrets. I wish the same for you.

Acknowledgments

This book never would have happened without the encouragement of Trish Newell and Mary Zgoda, who told me nearly as soon as I was diagnosed that I should write a book. My "posse" also includes Janie Harting (who designed the cover), Portia Dovel, Barb Lamoureux, Betsy Reece, Cindy Rieke and Katie Sosnowchik (who put on her formal book editing hat). Their feedback was insightful and their capacity to listen was limitless, during the publishing journey as well as the breast cancer journey. Speaking of the cancer journey, I want to thank my friend Pam Van Compernolle (the Warrior Princess). Pam lives each moment to the fullest, with zest and joy. She's my role model and hero.

I owe a huge debt of thanks to Teresa Forbes and Chris Christen, my editors at the *Omaha World-Herald*. Chris invited me to write the series of essays that turned into this book. Teresa helped me shape the series and was a great sounding board.

I would also like to thank the folks at Creative Byline who provided some dead-on developmental editing and feedback on the early outline and sample chapters, and David Collins at WingSpan Press, for guiding me through the publishing process. Lisa Pelto at Concierge Marketing and Jeff Beals, author of *Self-Marketing Power*, provided some great feedback as I was deciding to make the leap. And I probably wouldn't have made the leap if not for Kim Mickelsen, Bozell's resident social media goddess.

This book would have much less to offer if it weren't for four remarkable doctors: my general surgeon, Tim Kingston, M.D.; my family doctor, Gordon Moshman, M.D.; my oncologist, Gamini Soori, M.D.; and my plastic surgeon, Chester Thompson, M.D. Not only did they make my cancer adventure a largely positive one, but they graciously agreed to let me include them in this book, and I hope you enjoy their insights. I'm still knocked out by how generous they were with their time, and I will always be grateful to them, for their compassionate treatment and for making this book a better resource.

I would like to thank you, because if you're reading this you have purchased the book or at least considered it. I hope you find it helpful.

And first, last and always, I would like to thank my husband Bruce. I couldn't have asked for a better partner on this (or any) adventure.

Table of Contents

The phone call every woman dreads. The elephant in the room. Learning about my diagnosis—I had never heard of ductal carcinoma in situ or stage 0 cancer and thought cancer only came in stages 1 through 4. How a business trip after getting the news was actually a welcome distraction. Why the timing was not wonderful. How my DCIS was initially discovered, and the one thing I would have done differently out of this whole experience. The calm before the storm.

Reframing my "cancer belief system." What it was like getting the mastectomy recommendation from the first oncologist, and why getting a second opinion felt so urgent. Dealing with grief on different levels. Listening to my inner voice and canceling a trip home. How I came to terms with getting a mastectomy for a stage 0 cancer, which initially struck me as way too drastic. My "aha!" moment.

The new elephant in the room. Keeping track of all those doctors' appointments. Meeting my plastic surgeon for the first time. How Bruce and I took turns coping with our fears. Gearing up for the "Big M." Using music to drown out the undercurrent.

A welcome visit from friends. My amazing surgeon. The smuggled cooler and the zonked-out guard. My "dream team."

Chapter 4: Surgical Drains and the Well-Dressed Woman: Recovering from Mastectomy 57

What the timeline was like for activities such as showering, driving and exercising. What it was like going back to work. Those pesky surgical drains. Post-surgical exercises and worries about unlocking my armpit. How it was different at one, two and three weeks. Why shopping for clothes before I had my range of motion back probably wasn't the best idea. The great "cancer swag." How difficult but important it is to just rest and relax.

Chapter 5: My $83,000 Remodeling Project 71

Four and a half months after the combination mastectomy/first-stage reconstructive surgery, I had my stage-two reconstruction surgery combined with augmentation/lift of the other breast. What the surgeries were like, and how recovery differed this time. What it was like to go through nipple reconstruction surgery and getting the color tattooed in. What it cost when this was all said and done. The unexpected emotions that surfaced when it was finally over.

Chapter 6: How I Spent My Summer Vacation: Coping and Support 85

How this adventure was like a summer vacation. My husband's "tour of duty." "Underwear therapy." Friends and family and how do you talk about this to those who are not either one. Coping with the Flag Wavers and All About Me's. How things have changed in the way we communicate about cancer. Why I leaned on humor. To hug or not to hug? Our responsibilities as patients. How cancer became an unlikely muse and I started writing poetry again after a nearly 20-year absence. Pink ribbon activist or pink ribbon fatigue?

Q&A with my "Dream Team;" their perspectives and opinions on diagnosis and treatment. What women ask most often and what are some misconceptions about this diagnosis. What do those tingling and burning sensations mean after surgery. Who does and doesn't benefit from physical therapy. What are the different reconstructive options. What is AlloDerm® and why did my plastic surgeon use it. How do chemotherapy and radiation affect your reconstruction choices. Who is a candidate for immediate reconstruction and who is not. How should we communicate with each other.

"Warrior Princess"

Chapter 1:

What Did You Say I Have Again?

It's the phone call every woman dreads, and mine came on Wednesday, April 2, 2008. It was my turn to get breast cancer. I used to wonder how I'd handle it; now I wouldn't have to wonder anymore.

It was a jolt but I can't say it came as a complete surprise. Not because I have a family history or anything, which I don't, but because so many women are being diagnosed with breast cancer it almost seems like a rite of passage. But as rites of passage go, it's more like the first time you borrow your parents' car as a teenager and wreck it than getting your driver's license. It's one of those clubs no one wants to join.

As soon as my family doctor, Gordon Moshman, said the word "cancer" my brain started spinning like a hamster on a wheel and I grabbed the first thing I could find to write notes on. I knew I'd never remember the conversation. Dr. Moshman told me immediately that my particular "brand" of cancer, ductal carcinoma in situ or DCIS, was not life-threatening. Then he tossed out a lot of 50-cent words like "comedo" and "micropapillary" and I scribbled furiously along, trying to guess at the spelling.

He explained that DCIS is often successfully treated with breast-conserving surgery followed by radiation. So far, so good. Then he added that mastectomy has the best outcome, virtually guaranteeing a cure. I said that sounded pretty drastic for a non-life-threatening cancer. He said we'd talk and set up an appointment for the following Monday.

Dr. Moshman broke the news the night before I left on a

business trip for an annual engineering awards banquet in New York. He wasn't trying to be sadistic and ruin my trip; I had insisted on hearing the news before I left, because I'd be returning on Friday and didn't want the suspense hanging over my head for a second weekend (I had my biopsy the previous Friday, March 28). After he told me I had cancer I remember thinking, "Well, that's one way to get out of the cocktail party." One thing you'll find with cancer is it provides a perfect excuse to get out of doing things you don't want to do. Hey, there has to be a bonus in it somewhere.

After hearing the news, I would rather have stayed home but in a way I was glad to have the trip to distract me. I had to pack and make sure my dress still fit and finish all the other chores attendant on travel. But I also had to tell my husband Bruce. He was downstairs working out on the elliptical and wanted me to interrupt him, so I did. I said I do have cancer but it's not life-threatening and he was pretty calm, which was great. If he had freaked out at that moment, I might have too.

Bruce was probably just happy I told him anything. Leading up to the diagnosis, I hadn't been the best about relaying the news to him. I didn't tell him when I flunked the first mammogram because I wanted to spare him in case the second one turned out okay. When it didn't and they recommended a biopsy, I told him but I didn't win any style points. I was trying to figure out how to break the news when he told me after work one night that one of his colleague's wives needed a biopsy. I thought, "Great, here's my opening," and blurted, "I need a biopsy too."

I've never been very (or any) good at preamble. It might be good to preface news like this with, "I need to tell you something," or "We need to talk," something to at least give the person a warning. Bruce calls it the "Here's your bumper" syndrome. Years ago, I had a fender bender in his vehicle while he was out of town. When he got back, I told him about it (again, minus any kind of set-up) and handed him a piece of his bumper.

I had fleetingly thought of not telling Bruce until I learned how the biopsy turned out but I knew that wouldn't be fair to either one of us. He deserved to know, and I deserved to have his support because we were entering the realm of the scary unknown. Mammograms are maintenance but biopsies are a whole other deal. He went with me that day and although I told him he didn't have to, I'm grateful he did. This was the first of many trips we'd make together on this adventure. We had no clue just how many there would be.

The biopsy experience turned out to be quite educational. Like so many things about cancer you don't know until you get there, I didn't realize I had a choice when it came to biopsies. When I flunked the second mammogram, they called me back to the radiologist right away, who showed me the area of concern and recommended a biopsy as the next step. The radiologist told me I could choose a stereotactic biopsy or an excisional biopsy, also known as a wire localization. She said the excisional biopsy involved outpatient surgery and the stereotactic procedure was less invasive, so I arranged for one without doing any homework.

I really wish I had asked around before agreeing to that. I didn't talk to any women who've had either kind of biopsy. I didn't give Dr. Moshman a vote. I just told him I wanted the stereotactic biopsy.

If I could have done one thing differently out of this entire cancer experience, it would have been to skip the stereotactic procedure and go straight to the wire localization/outpatient surgery I ended up having anyway to remove the cancerous tissue. If my other breast ever goes bad I'm going to insist on it.

I know pain is subjective and we all have different thresholds, but the stereotactic biopsy hurt like hell. I found out later that a friend endured the same procedure and had the same response. (She called it barbaric. I prefer medieval, but you get the drift.) My surgeon told me after I had both procedures that the list of women who were unhappy with the stereotactic biopsy is pretty long. I told him to add me to the list.

The setup for it wasn't particularly comfortable. I climbed up on an elevated table and lay on my stomach with my breast sticking through a hole. They placed it between a couple of X-ray plates and injected a local anesthetic. The position of my arms and head wasn't anywhere close to comfortable, and I couldn't move for 45 minutes or so while they used a mammogram to pinpoint the area where the needle should be inserted. There was so much handling and prodding of my breast that I felt like a dairy cow.

Then came some sudden, searing pain I can't even really describe, except to say it's the one time I came close to a 10 on that one-to-10 pain scale medical professionals always want you to use. I never have understood that scale. Is two a headache? Is four menstrual cramps? I have no idea. But this hurt. It was definitely a 10 on the yelp scale. *Dr. Susan Love's Breast Book* says it's similar to getting your ears pierced at a jewelry outlet (and that the device's inventor originally called it a "biopsy gun." That should be a big hint right there.) I didn't get my ears pierced that way so I can't speak to the similarity, but I can't help but think if it felt anything like my biopsy did, they'd go out of business.

The wire localization procedure includes outpatient surgery with either local anesthetic with sedation, or general anesthetic, which carries risks, and you do have a bit more of a scar. But if I had to do it over again, I'd take that option in a heartbeat.

I said as much in one of a series of essays I wrote about my cancer experience for the *Omaha World-Herald*, and it generated the most response of anything I wrote. Close to a dozen women e-mailed that like me, they would never choose the stereotactic biopsy again. Several told me it's the worst pain they ever experienced, one adding a qualifier that she is not a wimp. (This was a recurring thread in the e-mails I got from female readers. So many women, including me, feel the need to apologize for or qualify our pain or even our opinions. It's high time we stopped doing that.) The worst part is several women had doctors and/or nurses who pooh-poohed their concerns or their pain.

I should note that my radiologist and her team couldn't have been nicer during my procedure and did their best to comfort me while I was yelling "Ouch! Ouch! Ouch!" (I'm surprised I didn't let loose with a few choice cuss words. I might have been too startled to swear.) She even apologized, but a little advance warning might have helped. I didn't think to ask if it was going to hurt and they sure didn't think to tell me. One of the techs offered me a chair afterward because she said a lot of women feel like they're going to pass out. I declined the chair and didn't feel in any danger of fainting, but I definitely felt like I'd been through the wringer.

I know painful procedures are the only option in certain situations, and if I ever need one of them I hope to cowboy up. But we have a choice with this one.

Of the six essays I wrote for the *World-Herald*, my biopsy essay was the only one to draw a response from the medical community. Two doctors e-mailed me and said they were sorry I had a bad experience and that they usually are successful at minimizing pain. Both of them were pretty nice. One of them said he wished I hadn't told women to "run for the exits" if anyone recommended this procedure. Fair enough, but I stand by everything I said.

The most interesting feedback came from a third doctor. He didn't contact me directly; someone else shared it. I think I made it pretty clear that this was based on my personal experience, but this doctor said they need to do something about an article written by a woman giving bad medical advice, because women were now questioning his group's recommendations.

The person who shared this with me asked me if it was my article and I said yes. I couldn't resist adding an unsolicited editorial comment—that the doctor seemed more interested in defending the procedure than in responding to women's concerns, and that we have the right to ask doctors why they recommend one procedure over another.

The fourth doctor I heard from had a completely different response. He told me a colleague brought up my less-than-glowing review of this biopsy type and I braced myself, thinking, "Great, here we go again." But what his colleague actually said was, "We have to do better for our patients." I know which one I'd prefer as my healthcare provider.

Here's my take on it: If there are reasons for choosing the stereotactic biopsy over the excisional biopsy, fine, tell us what they are and we'll make our choice, just like we do with cancer treatment. And choosing between radiation and mastectomy seems like a somewhat larger issue than which biopsy to get.

I'm getting a bit ahead of myself here. All I knew at the time was that I was not a fan of this procedure. I wouldn't learn until I wrote about it several months later that some doctors do not care to be questioned. The good ones will welcome your questions and respond to your concerns. The other ones need to learn that "Because I said so" is not a valid model of patient care.

The experience was a real eye opener and I have no regrets for creating a bit of a skirmish. And here's why: A woman I know called me after my essays ran to tell me she had the stereotactic biopsy and it was a piece of cake. I told her I was glad to hear someone had a good experience with it, and I meant it. She said she was really scared because of my essay and I apologized. Then she said, "No, because of you I asked questions and they gave me more Lidocaine than they normally would." I say that not to pat myself on the back, but to point out how important it is to ask questions, which is something I completely neglected to do going in. I chalk it up to a learning experience and hope others can learn from my mistake.

So, biopsy/nascent learning experience behind me—I was now an official member of the pink ribbon tribe. All in all, this bad news seemed to have quite a bit of good news attached. I mean, if you have to hear the word "cancer," it's best to hear "not life-threatening" in that same sentence. At this point, I felt pretty lucky, all things considered.

But trust me, no matter how early stage it is, hearing the "c" word is a shock. One minute you're brushing your teeth and thinking your usual random thoughts, and the next minute the realization hits you—"Wow, I have cancer." It definitely becomes the elephant in the room. It might not be poking you with its trunk at every conscious moment, but it's not leaving the room either and it does take up a good-sized chunk of psychic space.

When I got to New York, elephant serenely trailing behind me, my boss, Nancy, was also at the banquet and she knew I had been waiting to hear the results. She said she was sorry I had to show up for this event after getting that news, but I told her I was glad for the distraction. The banquet was as peacefully boring as ever, and oddly comforting. It was good to visit with the people I only see at these events. But my perspective was different. I looked at the bottles of wine on the table and wondered if I could have wine with dinner now or ever again—just one of the many things I did not know as I got ready to embark on this journey. How much would my life and my habits need to change? I decided one glass would be safe.

I did use the news as an excuse for getting out of the post-banquet cocktail party, and as I said before, cancer is a pretty good one. I'm not the schmoozing type even though I'm in public relations, so I was pretty content to go to my room and watch *The Office*. I found that as long as I was focused on something, like having a conversation or watching TV, the elephant stayed quietly in the corner. When I was in the shower or otherwise alone with my thoughts is when it started to stir.

I attended all the meetings with editors I had set up for our engineering experts the next morning, and again, it was good to have something to focus on but my mind was starting to wander. I felt like part of me was detached, watching myself go through the motions and seeing the elephant out of the corner of my eye. There's a small part of you that wonders if anyone else can see it, and for the most part they can't. But a colleague from our New

York office told me later, after I told him what was going on, that I had seemed pretty quiet.

When I got home Bruce and I were able to go about our usual business, but the elephant was starting to follow us around. I went to the grocery store and all the checkouts had little donation cartons for breast cancer. I remember wondering if this meant I could take money out now.

A big item on our "diagnosis to-do list" that first weekend was calling our family and friends. Our family calling tree was pretty short and had recently gotten shorter. My dad died suddenly at 76, three days after surgery, on February 21, 2008. I flunked my mammogram three weeks to the day later, on March 13. Which was kind of funny in the cosmic sense, because after Dad died, I remember thinking, "Well, my parents are both gone—not too much else can go wrong now." That type of comment is practically an invitation for fate to hand you something, and it sure did.

I was discovering all over again what a shape-shifter grief can be. It takes a different trajectory every time. Bruce's dad Duane died when he was 56. I was 28 then and Bruce was 27. When Duane died, I was a bit surprised and scared by how angry I felt. I remember seeing old people making their halting way into the grocery store and hating them for getting to stay when Duane didn't get the chance.

At the time I was working at a community mental health center and had access to professionals who helped me understand my feelings were normal. I thought grieving meant crying. I had heard of the various stages but never given it much thought. The grief workshop I attended was a bit anticlimactic though. I remember an exercise where we talked about all the things we'd do if we knew we were going to die soon, and the punch line was since that could be true, we better do them now. Yeah, I'll get right on that quitting my job and traveling thing. I'm sure the mortgage company will understand.

Bruce's older brother Brad died just over 10 years later, when he was 40. When Brad died, I wasn't angry but I woke up some mornings feeling like I weighed 400 pounds. I adored Brad. I could always count on him for perspective that I couldn't get from anyone else. There were times going through my cancer adventure when I wished I could talk to him, especially about the more absurd aspects. And as a former model booking agent in Los Angeles, he would have been all over the cosmetic surgery part of it.

I'm superstitious and I believe in the power of threes, so after losing Duane in 1984 and Brad in 1994, I was braced to lose another loved one in 2004. As it turned out, my mom didn't wait that long. She died October 1, 2003, after 50 years with Dad. I felt like one of those '60s-era Tiny Tears dolls, where you pull a string and they cry. I kept bursting into tears for weeks. This was grief as I understood it.

When Dad died, I missed him something awful but I also felt resigned to it more quickly than before. Maybe that's because when you hit your 50s you've finally figured out your loved ones are going to die, if they haven't already. I'd like to think I was more accepting of all of life's cycles, and in that sense maybe I was, but my acceptance skills were about to be sorely tested.

So Bruce and I were basically down to siblings. Our calling tree consisted of my brother Jerry and his wife Dawn in North Dakota, and Bruce's brother Jeff, sister Anita and her husband Jim in the Kansas City area.

And my dad's wife Bernice. She was Dad's childhood friend, married to his best friend Edwin, who had died of cancer some years earlier. Dad and Bernice were married in December 2004 and Dad moved back to his hometown in southwestern North Dakota. It was a nice way for him to come full circle and it was wonderful to not have to worry about him being lonely anymore. They had a great time in the three years they had together.

I felt the worst about calling Bernice and Jerry, because we were all still getting used to losing Dad and I felt like I was piling on. Bernice is in her 70s and has experienced enough bad news that she wasn't surprised to be handed more. And Jerry sounded worried, but as I kept telling him and everyone else, the cancer wasn't life-threatening and I like to have good news along with my bad news. I know that probably sounds a little too perky but I really believe that. I was grateful it wasn't stage 2 or 3. I also was sure I'd be like most women; they'd just cut the bad stuff out and I'd move on to radiation. I was already planning my schedule around it.

Some friends asked me if I felt like "Why me?" when I got the news and I really didn't. I mean, why not me? I just figured it was my turn. But that's not to say I didn't have a lot of WTF moments—if you don't know that particular online shorthand, it stands for "What The F*ck." Cancer hands you plenty of those— the big one, of course, is when you're diagnosed, but trust me, there are more to come.

Like many people who are newly diagnosed, I got online that weekend and started doing research. I kept thinking how I couldn't have done this 15 years ago. I love the Internet. It's a living breathing encyclopedia and conversation all rolled into one, right there at our fingertips. I mean, I can be watching a movie and want to know where it's filmed or what an actor's name is— and visit imdb.com and find out. Or trying to remember who said a certain quote, and there it is on quotations.com. It's a great tool for boomers with failing memories like me. I wasn't having quite as much fun looking up cancer statistics as I do movie trivia, but the instant access is great.

I read somewhere that the Internet is like sitting at a bar with a Ph.D. on one side of you and a drunk on the other, so I wanted to be a little careful on the medical research front, even though I knew I'd talk to Dr. Moshman about what I found. I visited webmd.com, mayoclinic.com and the Web sites for the American Cancer Society and National Cancer Institute. There seem to be a zillion Web sites discussing breast cancer in some way, shape or form, but these four seemed like they'd be among the most trustworthy.

I didn't go as far as researching tests and treatments because I didn't want too much detail at this point. I had never had surgery, never stayed in a hospital, never been diagnosed with a major illness. I was afraid I'd get too worked up if I got into too much technical detail. I like to know how things work and if possible, why they work that way, but I'm also squeamish about medical stuff (at least I used to be—more on that later). I just wanted to know what ductal carcinoma in situ was all about.

I've been faithfully getting mammograms since age 40 (I was diagnosed at 52), have a journalism degree and consider myself fairly knowledgeable about breast cancer. Yet I had never heard of DCIS and didn't know there was such a thing as stage 0 cancer, which is how DCIS is classified—I thought cancer only came in stages 1 through 4. I have since talked to two healthcare PR pros who had never heard of it either.

I found out I was certainly in good company. More than 178,000 women were diagnosed with breast cancer in 2007, according to the National Cancer Institute. And according to *The Breast Cancer Survival Manual*, 20 percent of all newly diagnosed breast cancers are DCIS. So that's roughly 35,000 of us going, "I have ductal what? WTF!"

Everything I saw online confirmed what Dr. Moshman told me. The good news about DCIS is that it's confined to the milk ducts ("in situ" means "in place"). Because it hasn't spread to other areas of the body, all the sources I looked at agreed that it's very treatable, with breast-conserving surgery and radiation often providing successful results. But you do need to treat it, or it can become invasive. And yes, they also mentioned the big bad "M" word, but I just figured that's not me.

We all make different choices, and I know some women say let's just get rid of the problem, remove the breast and move on, particularly women with a strong family history. Some women even opt for the bilateral mastectomy as a precaution. Women I've talked to who have done that told me they'd always be waiting for the other shoe to drop, and they didn't want to live like that. I could only think about one breast at a time and I wanted to keep it, so I latched on to radiation as my preferred option pretty quickly. There's no wrong choice here—just our choice.

I also went out and bought a pile of books, and this was another example of cancer providing a perfect excuse to be more of who you are. I love books and have way too many of them. This was a chance to add to my collection.

My survivor friend Pam was a great guide as I was trying to figure out what I should do and what I needed to know, including which books were most likely to be helpful. She's a teacher and I'm a writer and we share that inclination to research. She recommended *Dr. Susan Love's Breast Book*, *The Breast Cancer Survival Manual*, by John Link, M.D., and *Nordie's at Noon*, about four young Kansas City women battling breast cancer who became friends.

Like them, Pam lives in the Kansas City area and is way too young to be going through this. She's not even 40 yet, and just found out her breast cancer came back as stage 4. Nothing I went through can compare to what Pam is going through. But if anyone can face down this monster, it's Pam. She has gotten amazingly good results from her chemo and radiation so far and my money is on her. She has the face of a beauty queen and the heart of a lion.

I had no symptoms and no lumps, which I learned is typical. According to *The Breast Cancer Survival Manual*, 80 percent of DCIS cases are discovered through routine mammograms (I talked to an oncologist later who estimated it at more like 90 percent), which is how they found mine. It showed up as a tiny cluster of specks in my left breast. I couldn't even see them until they showed me a blown-up image. It looked like one of those satellite shots of the earth with clouds swirling over it, with a tiny smattering of bright white specks in one area. Thank God for young radiologists with good eyesight.

This was my first digital mammogram. A nurse told me later that they've noticed a huge jump in breast cancer detection since they started using them. Going through the mammogram itself was no different from the previous version that used film, but the process was a bit handier; the digital format allowed the technician to see right away if she'd need to get more views.

Nearly every time I have a mammogram I think of Ellen DeGeneres. Years before her talk show, she had a sitcom that had some truly inspired physical comedy moments. One of them was when she went in for a mammogram. She was fooling around with the equipment before the technician got there, and got her hand stuck in the vise. I've told that story to mammogram technicians more than once. If I ran a clinic, I'd have that scene playing on a loop. (I've never fooled around with the equipment myself.)

It seemed a bit late to look up risk factors for DCIS at this point, but I was curious. Mayoclinic.com says the risk factors for DCIS are the same as for invasive breast cancer—age, family history, genetic mutation, never being pregnant or having a late first pregnancy.

Alcohol wasn't on their list but the link between alcohol and breast cancer has been all over the media. In fact, while we were in the waiting room before one of my surgeries, Dr. Nancy Snyderman was on *The Today Show* saying the conventional drink-a-day ceiling for women was not safe, according to a recent study. Great. Just take me out behind the barn and shoot me and get it over with.

Here's the thing about me. I never met a glass of champagne I didn't like, and I like wine with dinner and mimosas with Sunday brunch. I believe good food and drink are two of life's great joys.

In terms of alcohol consumption, I'm somewhere in the middle. I'm not a role model, but I'm not a dire warning either. I know women who should have had full chest replacements and liver transplants by now based on their alcohol consumption, yet they're cancer-free. I know other women who have never had a drink and had breast cancer.

I did get carried away from time to time when I was younger, and more recently at a Nebraska-Texas football game. For the record, the recent crackdown on skybox alcohol at Memorial Stadium, where the Huskers play home games, is *not* my fault.

I've learned how to dial it down but I don't plan to give up alcohol completely. Someone once asked Julia Child the secret to her long life and she said, "Red meat and gin." My kind of gal!

It's quite possible my wayward youth contributed to my cancer to some extent. It's also possible that it's just the luck of the cosmic draw.

Exercise and weight don't seem to be the risk factors for breast cancer that alcohol is, but we've all heard about them with regard to general health and I'm somewhere in the middle on those fronts too. I don't have any grand designs other than being able to carry my own groceries when I'm 65. I'm no workout queen but I can lift 40 pounds of water softener salt in and out of the car and help move furniture.

Now that I was diagnosed with cancer, I started thinking about the overall state of my health. I was probably better off getting diagnosed now than five years earlier. When we hit our late 40s Bruce and I decided it would be a good idea to get in better shape for our senior years. And Dr. Moshman had started lecturing me about creeping weight gain because I started hauling another 10 pounds to every physical.

Dr. Moshman is quite trim—he probably weighs the same as he did in medical school. In fact, he's a colonel in the Army Reserve and on a recent deployment to Iraq, one of his tasks aside from surgery and exams was to help soldiers get in shape.

But back to unfit me. During one annual exam he asked me to what I attributed my weight gain. I said, "That would be eating and drinking." He laughed. I said, "What?" And he said most people aren't that honest. I just thought it was obvious. And besides, think about it. The one person who will know your underactive thyroid story is total B.S. is your doctor. I wish it would turn out to be like the movie *Sleeper* and they'd find out that steak and butter and alcohol are really good for you, but in the meantime, you might as well be honest. Your body won't lie for you in any case.

Enjoying life and being healthy may not be mutually exclusive for you, but I've had to find a balance between my vices and my health. Bruce and I have even talked about how if we knew we were terminal we'd crank some of our bad habits back up and maybe add some new ones.

Anyway, after we'd had the creeping weight gain talk for the second or third time, I asked Dr. Moshman if there was a diet he'd recommend. The South Beach Diet was getting a lot of attention at the time. He didn't recommend any; he just said you can't eat a wheelbarrow full of potatoes. True, but my efforts at portion control were not working; I needed structure. So Bruce and I went on the South Beach Diet—in Nebraska—in January—when all I wanted was a big bowl of stew and a nice Guinness to stave off the cold. I've since made my peace with eating salads in January but if you live in a cold climate like I do, you may want to take up dieting in July or August.

But it worked—we each took off about 30 pounds. We've gained some of it back but we're still in a lot better shape than we were five years ago, and we also got into the habit of exercising and actually liking it. On Valentine's Day last year we started our day working out at the St. Paul Hotel. But then we walked right over to Mickey's Diner for giant omelets with bacon and sausage. You don't want to get too carried away with this health thing.

So as I was taking stock, I was hoping that my semi-good, semi-regular habits would help me get through surgery and radiation. I knew I wouldn't need chemotherapy and I was very grateful for that because I've heard how grueling it is, but I've heard radiation can make you really tired. I figured being in halfway decent shape going in couldn't hurt.

When I look back on it, that first weekend after getting the news was like the calm before the storm. I did enough research to satisfy my curiosity but not enough to gross myself out. I wasn't eaten up with guilt over anything I might have done. We puttered around and watched a couple of movies to distract us from the elephant in the room. We called our family and friends and I managed to convince them and myself that I was lucky. "It's-cancer-but-it's-not-life-threatening" was practically my mantra.

We were scheduled to see Dr. Moshman on Monday to learn about our next steps, which we assumed would be surgery followed by radiation. This was before we realized how cancer can hand you a 180-degree turn in no time flat. We hadn't boarded the emotional roller coaster called cancer yet, but we were approaching the ticket gate.

Chapter 2:

The Decision Roller Coaster

It was official—I had DCIS. Now what? The next step was scheduling surgery to remove the offending tissue. We went to see Dr. Moshman the Monday after I got back from New York, April 7, so we could get this party started.

Dr. Moshman was my initial and primary contact. I was surprised to learn so many people I know don't have a family doctor, and if you do not, I urge you to find one. Bruce and I have been seeing him for about 15 years and I can't imagine going through this without him.

Dr. Moshman's first step was setting me up with Dr. Tim Kingston, a general surgeon he works with a lot. I trust Dr. Moshman but he doesn't editorialize much, so it was comforting to have his nurse Bridget tell me how much Dr. Kingston's patients like him. If you want to know if a doctor is any good, ask a nurse.

Bridget and Dr. Moshman's other nurses, Kathy and Pam, were all wonderful during this adventure but Bridget got me off to a great start. Contemplating surgery for the first time can be a little scary no matter what, not to mention a) it's cancer and b) it's in such a personal area. I eventually got used to whipping the girls out for inspection by someone or other on a weekly basis but there were times I really wished something was wrong with my arm or leg.

I got to have another new adventure during this visit—a pre-surgery EKG. So far I had had two mammograms, my first chest

X-ray and the lovely stereotactic biopsy. The new experiences were piling up.

We met Dr. Kingston for the first time on April 16 and as promised, both of us really liked him. He didn't get too technical; he's very intuitive and takes his cue from patients in terms of how much to say. I didn't want too much detail about surgery, thank you. He did say that the surgery should achieve good cosmetic results. That aspect hadn't even occurred to me so it was nice to hear.

We set up the surgery for April 25. I was nervous, but ready to get it over with so I could move on to radiation. My cancer belief system was becoming pretty firmly entrenched.

The surgery goes by various names depending on which doctor you talk to or which book you read—wide excision, lumpectomy or partial mastectomy. No matter what you call it, the goal is to remove the cancer while leaving your breast intact so I like the phrase "breast-conserving" surgery. I don't think lumpectomy seems quite accurate, since DCIS is so early stage there's no lump to remove. Second, I'm not a particular fan of the "M" word and would rather reserve its use for the real deal. To me, "partial mastectomy" is kind of like "jumbo shrimp."

As I mentioned earlier, my surgery would be immediately preceded by a wire localization, where they insert a wire into your breast via a needle. The wire guides the surgeon to the area of bad cells, since there is no visual cue like a tumor.

This particular part of the adventure stands out for me because of the inordinate amount of time it took to get the wire localization procedure, and the interesting cast of characters. We had to check in at the building where I'd have the outpatient surgery, then go to a different building for the wire localization. This turned out to be a group event because another woman was having the same procedure. She and her husband and Bruce and I traipsed through a maze of hallways with our hospital guide. It was a pretty long trek, made longer by the fact that this woman talked absolutely nonstop and I'm dead serious. She was like a Chihuahua after four or five espressos. Bruce and I trailed along behind them as far as we could.

When we got to the clinic where they did the wire localization, they took me to a ladies' only waiting room and left Bruce in a huge outer waiting room. They were running behind that day and I was trapped in that room for more than two hours, including an interruption by a fire alarm. They actually thought they might have to evacuate the building. At that point, I did go and sit with Bruce for awhile in the big waiting room. I figured if I had to wander around outside in a hospital gown I wanted to at least be with my husband.

For the life of me I don't know why I didn't bring an iPod or a book. I can't be in an airport without a book, and this big, busy facility resembled an airport, delays and all. And you know how most people are pretty much in "the zone," but there's that one loudmouth yakking on the cell phone in an extra loud voice? We didn't have that exactly, but we did have the woman who had accompanied me on the five-mile hike.

This woman not only had a bad case of verbal diarrhea, she also had an opinion on everything from surgery to my socks. I had decided I was going to find some way to amuse myself and own this experience, so I had a big pair of smiley face socks on. She pointed at my feet and said, "They told us to take off our socks!" Great—loud *and* a hall monitor. Nobody told me my first-ever surgery was going to be a trip back to junior high. I kept the socks on.

The wire localization already was not my idea of a good time; unless it's an underwire bra, I don't think the words "wire" and "breast" go together all that well. What was worse, my "companion" turned into an honest-to-God nightmare. She relished telling everyone who came in they had no idea of the hell she and I would be going through. This was another of many lessons I was about to learn regarding breast cancer—namely, that some people share cancer horror stories the same way others share childbirth horror stories.

For whatever reason, this woman made it her mission to scare the daylights out of everyone in that waiting room. After she had everyone sufficiently frightened of all things breast-related, she moved on to vaginal biopsies and how it was the most excruciating pain you could possibly experience. It's just too bad the rest of us were so polite and someone didn't tell her to shut the f*ck up.

The silver lining to this cloud was the kind lady who talked to me after the woman with the nonstop mouth finally left. I was completely cowering in the corner by this time and I'm sure I looked like I wanted to crawl under the chair. She told me she had found that it's best to just stay in your own little bubble and ignore what everyone else has to say.

When they called the kind lady to get her mammogram, she came over and put her hand on my shoulder and said, "Remember, stay in the bubble." I've found that the cancer adventure offers many such moments of kindness, and I hope that I have managed to repay some of them, through my writing if nothing else.

I was terrified of the wire localization, not just because of what my nightmare companion said, but because I kept thinking, "Okay, if the stereotactic was *less* invasive, what the bleep is *this* going to be like?" I was worked up into a pretty good lather by the time I finally got in for the procedure. I got even frothier when they said I wouldn't get a local anesthetic, which contradicted what I had heard earlier. I kept telling myself that at least the pain shouldn't last too long. Bless the nurse who read my face and told me it's like a needle stick for a blood draw, and she was right. The moral of that story is to listen to the nurses, not the waiting room freaks.

This procedure was generally more comfortable. It was like a seated mammogram, except the paddles or plates or whatever they call those things they tighten over your breast have holes in them to accommodate the needle. It really was a piece of cake.

And now that my brain was no longer ordering me to assume the fetal position, I was able to find some humor. With a syringe sticking out of my chest, all I could think about was the cocaine overdose scene in *Pulp Fiction*, when John Travolta jammed a needle full of adrenaline into Uma Thurman's chest. I asked the team if they had ever seen the movie. Three of them didn't get the reference but one laughed, for which I was grateful.

It got even more "Pulp Fictionish" from there; to keep the wire from being bumped out of position, they placed a Dixie cup over it and taped it to my chest, then arranged the robe over it, I guess so as not to scare any passers-by. Now I really was having a flashback, because I actually dressed up like the post-overdose Uma Thurman character one Halloween, and we secured a dog-vitamin syringe to my chest using, you guessed it, tape and a Dixie cup cut in half.

I was glad to have pop culture trivia to keep my brain occupied while being wheeled over to the other building for my first surgery. Especially since they also seemed to misplace Bruce and didn't appear too concerned that he'd be able to find me one building away through a labyrinth of hallways. I kept asking to wait and they assured me they'd find him. I think they were running so late they just wanted to get me out of there.

The cool thing about showing up for surgery was seeing my name on the white board. "Hey," I told the orderly. "It's just like Grey's Anatomy!" (Did I mention I have a lot of pop culture trivia lodged in my head and it takes next to nothing to amuse me? This comes in pretty darn handy when you have cancer.) The bad thing is my husband had no clue they had taken me and I had no way to reach him. Thank goodness for the beautiful young tech who helped me get onto my gurney. She called Bruce on her cell phone for me; another act of kindness for which I was grateful.

I was also really grateful for Dr. Kingston and his team. There's a real knack to putting people at ease before they go into surgery, and they all have it. All of his nurses were great, and he's in a league of his own. He just radiates calm. He comes in and rubs your arm or holds your hand and it's amazing how much a little thing like that helps. He adjusted my sheets and told me he liked my socks. (Take that, Motor Mouth Hall Monitor!)

In case anyone reading this is a surgery virgin like I was, I learned a couple of things that may be helpful. Since I'd never had surgery, I wasn't sure how it would affect me. They put the routine medication for nausea in my IV but it wasn't enough. I yakked in the recovery room and again on the way home, and almost did it again the next morning when I tried reading the paper. It was like really intense motion sickness. So here's my helpful hint, learned the hard way: talk to your doctor about getting that motion sickness patch they put on your neck.

Another big one—leave those little sterile strips over your incision alone. For some reason, after two days I decided I should just start yanking them off. Not smart. I caught on and stopped after the second one. The blood bubbling up was a bit of a clue. Luckily, there wasn't much.

I also learned that you probably shouldn't get on a motorcycle two days after surgery. Bruce and I went out for a short, hour-long ride on his Harley and I felt every bump. That advice probably seems like common sense, but I thought I'd throw it in for anyone who might be as ignorant as I was. Pam warned me about getting on a motorcycle but we did that before I got her e-mail.

The surgery wiped me out a lot more than I expected. I had it done on a Friday and figured the weekend should be plenty of recovery time, but when I went back to work Monday I was pooped. The pain was less than minimal and I didn't need any of the pain pills they sent home with me; I was just really wiped out. I went home and took a nap and still went to bed by 8:00 p.m. I guess it takes the anesthesia a few days to work its way out of your system.

It took a few days to get the results. As I mentioned earlier, I assumed that I was going to be done after this surgery and moving on to radiation, which I had learned a little about. Dr. Kingston explained that it would take five days a week for six weeks. He said he knew someone who scheduled it over her lunch hour after the initial visit, which takes longer because they're figuring out the coordinates. I had asked him about side effects and he said they were less than they would be if you were radiating a body cavity. I thought, "Hey, if I can get this done over my lunch hour that's not too bad." We had a trip home coming up in late May and I figured I'd start radiation after we got back. It all seemed quite tidy.

The thing none of us could know going in was that the tiny specks on my mammogram were just the tip of the iceberg. The surgery didn't catch all the cancerous cells, even though Dr. Kingston removed seven centimeters (2.75 inches) of tissue. With DCIS, doctors want what they call "clean margins." The conventional wisdom, which I've read about and heard from my doctors, defines clean margins as at least one centimeter. I was nowhere near that.

Not what I wanted to hear, but during our visit on May 2 Dr. Moshman told me it often takes two surgical procedures to get it all. Okay, this wasn't the end of the world and I didn't feel like I could see it from here, at least not yet.

So on to round two of surgery (the guide wire was no longer necessary). I could have opted for a mastectomy at this point but both Bruce and I thought it was worth another try.

We scheduled the second surgery for May 16. In the meantime, I had my regularly scheduled physical with Dr. Moshman on May 14. We ended up just talking since I had a visit from "my friend," as we used to say in grade school; that may be why I felt like I wanted to chew the poor man's head off.

Just about everything Dr. Moshman said struck me the wrong way that day. At one point, he said something about not needing radiation, which I instantly and wrongly interpreted to mean I needed a mastectomy. This was my cue to say something but instead, I clammed up. I gave Bruce an earful on the phone later though, and, unknown to me, Bruce called him. Before I knew it I had a voice mail at home from Dr. Moshman apologizing for not communicating very well. I felt like a huge jerk, so I left him a voice mail saying it takes two to communicate and I didn't hold up my end of the bargain either.

Here's the deal. Doctors are wonderful people. They're also brutally busy. They may not always perfectly pick up where you left off the time before. I'm impressed by how well all of my doctors usually did remember where we left off. I only had four doctors to keep informed of my decisions and sometimes I didn't even remember what I had said to whom. I don't know how they do it.

I do remember asking Dr. Moshman that day if he planned on recommending an oncologist and I know I had an edge to my voice. I was getting very impatient and had actually scheduled my own oncology consult for the following week, someone recommended by a friend. I was planning to get a second oncology opinion anyway, because I felt like I should for something this serious, but I was annoyed that he hadn't made a recommendation yet.

This is another weird thing about cancer. When you're grappling with this diagnosis, your mind is reeling and you sometimes feel like you have to do something *right now*. This process all seemed a bit too leisurely for me. Dr. Moshman was willing to take it one step at a time, but I was not.

And since cancer doesn't happen in a vacuum, I had other things going on at home and at work. Shortly after I got back to the office from New York, our assistant media relations coordinator gave me his notice. Joe had been with us for nine months. He is a wonderful young man, sweet and funny and smart but so quiet I told him once that sharing an office with him was like sharing space with a cat.

Joe is nothing like me in the "Here's your bumper" sense. After arriving at work that morning, he launched into the "We need to talk" preface. When he told me he was leaving us to go to law school, I started laughing. The timing was just too perfect. He planned to stay through the end of May, so I now had interviewing and hiring on my plate. I told him what was going on with me since I'd be missing a fair amount of work for all my appointments.

When May 16 rolled around, I felt better because I knew what to expect from surgery this time. The guide wire was no longer necessary so we didn't have to trudge between two buildings. Dr. Kingston was just going to remove more tissue and, I hoped, clear out all the bad stuff with margins to spare.

When he stopped by pre-op this time, he pulled the curtain aside and said, "I'm ba-ack," kind of like Jack Nicholson in *The Shining*. It was pretty funny. I asked if many women end up coming back and he said he and his team have a way of wearing out their welcome.

I was trying really hard not to think ahead to what would happen if this didn't work, but I couldn't help asking if he'd also do the mastectomy in case we didn't get it all this time. I was so ignorant going into this I didn't realize he did both types of surgery and was hugely relieved when he said yes. I didn't want to start over with someone else, especially since he has that "patient whisperer" way about him.

Pam had sent us a pair of his and her "F*ck Cancer" stocking caps (blue for Bruce and pink, of course, for me) so we took mine to surgery and Bruce took my picture in it. It was a huge hit with Dr. Kingston and his team. One of his nurses wanted to know how to get one for her aunt, who had just been diagnosed. When the nurse anesthetist showed up, the first thing she said was, "I want to see that hat!"

There was a little unintentional humor on my part when Dr. Kingston reached over to mark the surgery spot with an X. I asked him why he didn't do that the time before and as the words were leaving my mouth I realized that the Dixie cup and wire had been a fairly massive visual clue. Duh. He just looked over at Bruce like he was looking for help or maybe confirmation that I really was that dumb.

And as cool a veteran as I thought I was being with one whole surgery under my belt, my left leg started bouncing under the sheet after Dr. Kingston left, in spite of the drugs they gave me to relax. The only other time I've ever had that happen was when I was learning to ride a motorcycle. When I was practicing turns in the parking lot, my left leg was jumping like a Jack Russell. (I wonder why it's always my left leg?) Bruce told me later that my tongue was shaking when the nurse took my temperature. I couldn't tell and didn't even know tongues could shake.

Apparently they put me under a little deeper this time although I couldn't tell any difference. Dr. Kingston told me in pre-op that the time before I was napping but this time I would be sleeping. (Later on, I asked him what the difference was and he explained he used local anesthesia with sedation for the first surgery. He used general anesthetic for the second one because the local anesthetic might have distorted the boundaries of the tissue being excised. That wasn't an issue the first time because the guide wire was a direct road map.)

I actually stayed alert longer for this one—I saw the oxygen mask coming at my face before I zonked out. Whatever they give you sure works. Bruce, who really is a surgery veteran, had told me before that it's the best sleep you ever had. (We've joked since then that although he holds the lifetime record with eight surgeries, I hold the land-speed record having six in just over a year, including my gallbladder.)

Dr. Kingston came to see us while I was in recovery because Bruce missed him when he came out to let him know how I did. Bruce had asked if he had time to go get coffee and was told yes.

It was interesting because you could hear this ripple effect as he came in. I heard at least a couple of nurses saying, "Dr. Kingston's coming." It was kind of like when you're in line at a public venue and someone spots a celebrity and the whispers get passed down, but it was more than that. I was halfway expecting the curtains to billow open as he passed.

They gave me the anti-nausea patch this time and I was very happy to come around without throwing up. I was also happy to be able to walk to the car instead of being pushed in a wheelchair like I was the first time. We even went to our favorite Mexican restaurant for lunch. Bruce suggested it as kind of a joke and was shocked when I said yes and was able to eat, but after we got home I took a pretty lengthy nap.

I felt this surgery a bit more afterward. I didn't really feel any pain with the previous one, other than the aforementioned motorcycle bouncing. This time I could feel a little pain when I moved or stretched just right, but nothing that Tylenol couldn't fix.

I had the surgery on a Friday again, but this time I took Monday off and it helped because I took a three-hour midday nap instead of trying to drag my way through work. Napping would turn out to be a big part of my recovery strategy. I highly recommend it.

Prior to the second surgery, Dr. Kingston said you can still get reasonably good cosmetic results, and he did. I was impressed by what a good job he did for as much as he took out. From certain angles it almost looked normal. From other angles it looked kind of deflated but I'm at that age and stage of gravity where that wasn't such a departure from normal either.

I think it was during the follow-up visit after this surgery that I realized I still wasn't all that blasé about having my chest examined. I had gotten used to Dr. Kingston looking at the left one. All of a sudden he was looking at the right one and I asked him why. My comfort window, if you can call it that, didn't extend to the right side. He said he was checking for symmetry. And as I mentioned, it was pretty decent.

After the second surgery, I had clear margins but just barely— less than 1 millimeter compared to the desired 1 centimeter. Dr. Kingston thought I might be able to start radiation but said I should talk to an oncologist. As it happened, I had scheduled my first oncology consult just two hours after our appointment. And while Dr. Kingston did not say, "Go forth and radiate," Bruce and I took his comments as gospel and immediately called our family and friends.

Imagine our reaction when the consult, after reviewing my chart and taking a family history, said, "I know you don't want to hear this but I think you need a mastectomy." I felt like I had been sucker punched. Bruce told me later that I leaned back as far as I could while sitting on that tall examining table, like I was trying to get away. I was completely unaware of doing that.

For nearly two months I had been assuming that I was on the path to radiation, and I can't turn my emotions on a dime. I could not wrap my mind around something as drastic as a mastectomy for a stage 0 cancer.

Every alternative I brought up seemed to be a dead end. When I asked about radiation, the reply was it may or may not work but nothing works as well as steel. That remark didn't even register with me at first, but Bruce cringed. That's the type of thing you tell a medical student, not a patient who's hearing for the first time that she needs a mastectomy. This was not an intellectual exercise for me. Doctors need to be mindful there's a person attached to the breast.

I asked about Tamoxifen, which is a pill you take to prevent cancer from reoccurring if your cancer is estrogen-dependent like mine was, and was told I couldn't take it because of my fibroids. (I'll spare you the details on my fibroid history.) I felt like door after door was slamming shut. Bruce was sitting in the corner with his head pinging back and forth like he was watching a tennis match.

I also heard that I could try a third surgery but that it probably wasn't worth it because this oncologist thought I had a "diseased breast." I was too stunned to be angered by the tone of this conversation, but I became very angry later. Hello, can I at least have dinner and a drink first?

The absolute worst part was when this doctor recommended that I get magnetic resonance imaging (MRI), which the American Cancer Society now recommends as an adjunct test for women who are at high risk because of dense breast tissue or other factors. The MRI itself didn't seem like a bad idea, but this doctor brought it up in the context of whether a bilateral mastectomy would be indicated. Sucker punch number two.

At that point I finally grew a spine and said, "Hold on a minute—I'm just now hearing that I might need to lose one, and you're bringing up two?" Although most of this conversation is permanently seared into my head, I can't for the life of me remember how the doctor responded to that.

I was pretty numb by this time and dumbly agreed to set up an MRI, and then the doctor left. The whole process took about 20 minutes. I held it together until we got outside and then had a full-tilt meltdown. After comparing notes with friends later, I learned that the parking-lot meltdown is yet another cancer tradition.

Going back to work was out of the question. We had both driven to the oncologist's office and Bruce wasn't sure I'd be able to drive myself home. But after about 10 minutes of crying my guts out, I was calm enough to get home, although I started right up again after I got there.

I don't doubt for one second that this highly regarded doctor was driven by giving me the best possible outcome, but this tough love approach was not a good fit. As it turned out, Bruce wasn't comfortable with this doctor's blunt style either, but he didn't tell me how he felt until I told him I didn't think I was going back. He wanted to leave it up to me. (This was hard on him too. When we were newly married, he was in the Navy and I often tell people "we" were in the Navy because I definitely felt like I did a tour of duty as a spouse. It's the same with cancer. We were about six weeks into it and both of us had just been handed another huge WTF.)

The take-away here is that you're going to be spending a lot of time with your doctors and trust me, you need to feel comfortable with them. It doesn't matter how good the doctor is or how many happy patients he or she has; the relationship has to feel right for *you*. Don't feel guilty if you decide to choose a different doctor, no matter how highly the first one was recommended or by whom. This is your body and your life.

Since I'm recounting everything the oncologist said that I didn't like, it's only fair to mention that I said something unbelievably stupid. I actually said, "Why can't I just keep an eye on it and if it does turn into stage 2 cancer just deal with it then?" The doctor responded, "But why would you want to put yourself through that?"

I can see now how right that response was, especially in light of my friend Pam being in the fight of her life against the stage 4 monster, but at the time I was determined to find a way out. I was not even close to ready to accept what I heard.

The doctor did say one other thing I found pretty compassionate. I had asked how much time off I would need if I went through with the mastectomy, and the response was, "One week is good and two is even better. You don't get any points for being tough."

This was May 22 and it seriously was one of the worst days of my life. I had never gone from such a high to such a low in the space of two hours. Now I was getting up close and personal with the cancer roller coaster. I canceled the MRI I had set up. No way was I ready to deal with the possibility of having both breasts removed.

I was lying on the couch reeling when Dr. Moshman called. He asked me how I was and I said I've been better. His timing was uncanny; I actually wondered for a second if he was psychic. But he called because he had just gotten the lab results and wanted me to come in so we could talk. We set up an appointment for the next day.

The visit with Dr. Moshman on May 23 stands out for me

because of something he said. He told me if I were his wife he'd want me to get the mastectomy because he thought the risk of getting invasive cancer was just too high. He'd seen it happen before.

This stands in stark contrast to what Dr. Link says in *The Breast Cancer Survival Manual*. The book is an excellent resource, but the one clunker for me was when he said he finds it insulting to be asked what he'd do if the patient was his wife. His reasoning is that the question implies a different standard of care. Dr. Moshman offered his thoughts without my asking, and I found it comforting. I didn't decide on the spot I was up for it—far from it—but his concern meant the world to me then and it still does.

This moment is when I was reminded that cancer happens when you're making other plans. You may end up changing some of those plans as you come to grips with your decisions; the key is to listen to your inner voice.

I mentioned that my dad died in February, shortly before I was diagnosed. We had gone to his funeral on February 26; his graveside service was scheduled for May 26. Bruce and I planned to attend the ceremony and our twin nephews' high school graduation a couple of days earlier. When we planned the trip, we were still assuming my treatment would be radiation, and the trip would be a welcome break before starting it. I wanted to see my nephews graduate and while I can't say I looked forward to saying goodbye to Dad again, I wanted to be there for his 21-gun salute.

The first clue I might need a mastectomy came a couple of days before we were supposed to leave. Here's where that inner voice comes in and I didn't listen to mine right away. After my initial meltdown, I kept saying I'm fine, we have to go home but suddenly dreaded the trip. My stoic act collapsed when I burst into tears at the restaurant where Bruce and I were having lunch on our way to see Dr. Moshman. Bruce just looked at me and said, "You're not ready for prime time." And I wasn't. I needed that week to calm down and try to get an appointment for a second opinion. My brother and the rest of my family understood, and I have no regrets.

I'm not saying you should cancel all your plans. But you do need to give yourself time, less to think than to not think, because your mind will race like a hamster on a wheel. You may find your stillness through prayer or meditation; I rely on music but I did occasionally pray for calm or strength or both. Friends and family also prayed for me, and their prayers were most welcome.

You ultimately want to get to the place where you're not second-guessing your decision. Your doctors will give you their best counsel but it's your choice, and it's a lonely one. You'll know when you get there because the churning will stop.

I mentioned feeling some urgency about getting a second oncology opinion. A good friend, Doug, had recommended a different oncologist, Dr. Gamini Soori, as soon as I was diagnosed, and he became more insistent after the mastectomy recommendation. Doug kept telling me about Dr. Soori's credentials and I kept putting him off. I figured I'd eventually see whoever Dr. Moshman recommended. But when I flipped out after the first consult, Doug told me how much his friends both liked Dr. Soori when he treated the wife for her cancer. "Like" was the magic word. I wanted in.

While we were waiting to meet Dr. Soori for the first time, I said, "Well, at least nothing can shock me now." Bruce lowered his voice and said, "I'm sorry; we're going to have to cut off your head." That cracked me up and I was mortified to be laughing in this hushed waiting room but I just couldn't seem to stop. I got up and walked over to the magazine rack to calm down and it worked for a few seconds but then it started bubbling up again. I felt like I was laughing in church. I finally stopped but it was one of those deals where knowing how inappropriate it is makes you laugh even more.

The difference in oncology consults was night and day. Dr.

Soori spent an hour and 20 minutes with Bruce and me during that first visit and reminded us we had options, which is exactly what I needed to hear.

Like the first oncologist, Dr. Soori recommended an MRI to catch anything the mammogram might have missed, but said that while they would look at both breasts he assured us that it was mainly a precaution; he said discovering cancer in both breasts is extremely rare. He asked if he could present my case to his team of oncologists and radiologists.

He also said he did have some concerns and asked me to keep an open mind. I told him I would and asked him if he would take me as his patient. I had looked over at Bruce at one point while Dr. Soori was talking and he just nodded. We could both tell he was the one.

At this point Dr. Moshman knew I had gone oncologist shopping again. I let him know I decided to stay with Dr. Soori, and he wasn't offended I found my own cancer doctor. When I had a moment of guilt and wondered if I shouldn't check out the group he would have recommended too, he let me off the hook. "There's such a thing as getting too many opinions," he told me.

I had the MRI on June 6. I had never had one before and had heard they can be really claustrophobia-inducing. I think unless you are claustrophobic in other situations, you'll be fine. The noise bothered me more than anything but it was bearable. It was a bunch of pounding that varied in frequency. I had headphones with music (Enya to be exact—I asked for classical but she didn't have any) and the technician would cut in every once in awhile to say, "This next sequence will last for six minutes. (THUMP THUMP THUMP) You're doing great." The whole thing took about half an hour.

It probably helped that I was on my stomach and looking down at the floor, so I didn't have that enclosed sensation like you might if you were on your back. It didn't feel like being stuffed inside a tube. The place where I had it done had a little mirror set up so you could look at a landscape print they had on the wall. It didn't really do anything for me but it was a nice touch. It reminded me of many years ago when "we" were in the Navy. The doctor I always saw at the Jacksonville Navy medical facility for my Pap smear had a poster of a kitten on the ceiling above the exam table that said "Hang in there, baby." Pretty cornball but it's the thought that counts.

Dr. Soori told me we're at the point with MRIs now that we were with mammograms 20 years ago in terms of frequency and expense. And they are expensive—mine was just under $4,000. My insurance carrier did pay for it but enforced a 10-day waiting period, so be sure you work within your insurance carrier's guidelines.

After the MRI, I did something that another cancer survivor friend had advised me to do. She's a private person so I won't use her real name. I'll call her Audrey. She's a five-year survivor and like Pam, she was a great mentor during this adventure.

Audrey said she always used to treat herself to something after she reached a milestone in treatment. So I used that as an excuse to go to a nearby coffee shop called The Village Grinder for lunch before I headed back to work. It's attached to a bookstore called The Bookworm in a cute little shopping center and is surviving quite well even though Starbucks is a short walk away. Come to think of it, The Bookworm is Omaha's last surviving independent bookstore. I hate to admit I'm part of the problem; I've gone the Amazon route for the most part, but I did buy my stack of breast cancer books there.

To give you an idea of The Village Grinder's vibe, I went there for lunch with a friend once and someone pulled up in a Smart Car. They're still pretty rare in Omaha, and the women baristas and customers came outside to coo over it like it was a new baby. It reminded me of when I had my Camano Z28, which was a magnet for men young and old; and later my Toyota FJ Cruiser, which also drew a lot of men, as it was one of the first in Omaha. (That was an accident; I'm not a trendsetter or gearhead but I tend to like some of the same cars guys like. And the FJ was a total impulse buy; when I took my Highlander in for an oil change, I saw one on the lot and I was smitten. Did I mention I'm shallow?)

But I digress. The MRI wasn't particularly stressful but after I finished, I did have one of those "Stop the world, I want to get off" moments. It was great to just sit for awhile and watch the world go by in this cozy little coffee shop before heading back to work. A feeling of peace washed over me and I was thankful to Audrey for what wouldn't be the last time.

I felt some much-needed calm after talking to Dr. Soori but the roller coaster was still swooping and diving. (I should have asked for a patch.) I'd find myself going through several stages of grief in as many minutes, from denial to anger to bargaining and back again, and also some plain old flip-flopping. I'd do radiation. No, I'd play it safe and get the mastectomy. Just what the hell *would* I do? I already had one doctor tell me what to do, and I didn't want to hear it. I had my family doctor, whom I like and respect, tell me what he hoped I'd do, and I didn't want to do it. Now I had a third one tell me it was going to be my choice, which is all I want in life, and I wasn't sure I could handle it. I still wanted radiation and I just couldn't figure out how I was going to choose a mastectomy if it came to that.

While I was wrestling with this decision, I noticed how time goes through the same weird stretching-out process it goes through when you're grieving. Ten minutes feels like an hour, and an hour feels like a day. And a corollary to that is that your attention span is shot. Sometimes I felt like my train of thought lasted for all of two seconds before being completely derailed.

I know cancer is big enough to inspire these reactions all by itself—I have enough friends who have ridden that roller coaster—but I think part of it is that I was still grieving over my dad. I missed him every day and facing this big decision made it worse. I only had a few weeks to grieve over him before the elephant called cancer showed up and started commanding all that psychic space.

Bruce and I would talk about whether my dad would want to be around for this adventure or not. Bruce didn't think he'd want to see his daughter have to go through this. I thought he'd rather be here than not. It would have been fun to compare medical notes with him, although with what he was facing I truly believe it was a blessing he got to go so quickly. They had discovered he had stage 4 rectal cancer and he was facing some pretty punishing treatment after he recovered from surgery. Instead, a pulmonary embolism took him out. He was walking down the hall with Bernice on one side and a nurse on the other and he just said "Oh," and was gone.

Dad used to say that when the good Lord was ready to call him home, he hoped He'd just yank his chain. God showed mercy on Dad by doing just that, and if you knew my dad you'd know how much he deserved it. You could hold a gun to his head to try to get him to say something bad about someone, and he couldn't do it. Whenever I get the urge to see the other person's side of the story, I blame him.

My emotions around Dad were still pretty raw but I also caught myself missing Mom a lot. It doesn't matter who you are or how old you are, if you feel any kind of sickness you want Mom. I was 47 when she died of colon cancer so I had five years to get used to it, but this brought it back big time. I could tell her stuff I could never tell Dad, and I found myself doing that now.

Some nights I'd lie awake missing both of them so much I felt an ache in my chest. I know how lucky I am to have my husband and the rest of my family and friends, but there's just something about Mom and Dad. Christopher Buckley wrote a book called *Losing Mom and Pup: A Memoir.* I haven't read the book yet, but I read an interview with him in *AARP The Magazine* where he said your parents are your ultimate protectors, and talked about the comfort you get from just knowing they're there. He said,

"They're like fire extinguishers mounted on the wall behind glass. You know if it really comes to it, you can break the glass. And now they're gone."

June 11 was Judgment Day—we were back in Dr. Soori's office to learn his opinion after reviewing the MRI results and consulting with his team. If you ever got called to the principal's office as a kid, this was a hundred times worse.

Unfortunately, his recommendation was the same as the first oncologist's. While the MRI was clear, he said I had too many specific risk factors for invasive cancer. Red flags included the large amount of cancer cells, the type of cells (they range from low to high in aggressiveness and mine, the cribriform type, is intermediate), and the fact that my breast tissue is dense, making it hard to see what's going on. The one area where he differed was in recommending that I start a daily Tamoxifen regimen for five years to protect the other breast. I was only too happy to comply with that part of it. Although Dr. Soori recommended the mastectomy, he told me he would support me if I opted for radiation and surveillance, as long as I understood the risks.

Like Dr. Moshman, Dr. Soori told me he couldn't do any better for me if I was a member of his own family. And like Dr. Moshman, he offered this perspective without being asked. I asked Dr. Kingston about this later when I was fact-checking something I was writing. I wanted to know what women ask him most often and he said he gets the "What would you do if I were your wife?" question a lot. I asked him if he found that insulting and he quickly said, "No, not at all." So I just as quickly explained it was Dr. Link's point of view, not mine.

I have never for one second thought that any of my doctors might try harder for a family member than he would for me. But I can tell you how reassuring it is to hear a doctor tell you this is what he'd do if cancer affected someone he loves. It's personal and human, and nice.

And it's funny, because although I have never asked a doctor that question, I have asked financial advisors where they put their own money. Which just goes to show you my priorities are completely messed up.

Naturally, Dr. Soori's recommendation wasn't what I wanted to hear. I wasn't sobbing my guts out like I did after the first consult, which was good because I prefer doing my crying in private, but I definitely needed the Kleenex Dr. Soori handed me. He acknowledged this by simply saying, "It's hard for a woman to lose her breast." Yes indeed. Some little corner of my mind was thinking, "Poor guy. This part of the job must suck." When I went to shake his hand as we were leaving, he hugged me instead. That was unexpected but very nice.

This was the first time I noticed the boxes of Kleenex strategically placed around his receptionist's area. I never noticed them before because I didn't need any. This time I needed a fistful. We set up a follow-up appointment in three weeks.

By the time we left Dr. Soori's office, I already knew what I had to do. Too many sharp minds were making the same recommendation.

The first oncologist had estimated my overall risk of getting an invasive cancer within five years at 50 percent. Dr. Moshman estimated 30 percent. The thing to remember about risk is that those numbers really only apply to groups. I figured my personal risk was more like zero or 100 percent—I'd either get it or not.

My "aha!" moment came when I finally remembered just how risk-averse I am in the rest of my life. Not only am I conservative when it comes to investing, I can't even stand the TV show *Deal or No Deal*. If you haven't seen it, it's the one where contestants bet on whether a suitcase they picked holds a million dollars. Bruce used to watch it sometimes and I had to leave the room every time. I'm not above mindless entertainment; I just couldn't take the stress. I've seen people turn down a quarter of a million dollars and I'm ready to fold the tent at $20,000. What made me think I'd want to gamble with my life?

Make no mistake, I was sad and I had every right to be, but it was the kind of sadness you feel when you've let go of something. I had known I might need a mastectomy for a good three weeks but I had been fighting it. I knew I wasn't going to fight anymore.

I slept better that night than I had in a long time, and the next morning I felt calm for the first time in weeks. I didn't spring out of bed happy by any means, but the churning in my head had finally stopped.

Chapter 3 :

To Mastectomy, and Beyond!

I don't want to imply that once I decided, facing the mastectomy was a walk in the park. I was at peace with my decision but it was still plenty scary. You can tell yourself all you want that it's just another body part, but there's something so deeply personal about having a mastectomy. I've had gallbladder surgery since then and trust me, they're nothing alike on the physical or emotional fronts. There's no equivalent of "Save Second Base" T-shirts for the gallbladder. As Bruce put it, they're messing with the playground.

Now that we knew I'd need a mastectomy and reconstructive surgery instead of breast-conserving surgery and radiation, Dr. Moshman's next step was setting me up with a plastic surgeon. He also consulted with Dr. Kingston, and recommended Dr. Chester Thompson. Dr. Kingston and Dr. Thompson often work together on breast cancer cases. Because I could undergo immediate reconstruction, first Dr. Kingston would perform the mastectomy and then Dr. Thompson would place the tissue expander as the first step in reconstruction. Dr. Soori told me you get very good results when they can work as a team that way.

I'm glad he told me that because it was just one of the many, many things I didn't know enough to appreciate at the time. Another one was the way Dr. Moshman coordinated my care and communicated with me about each next step. During this time there was a study in the news that said many women are not even told about their reconstructive choices before having cancer surgery. Nothing could have been further from my experience, and once again I felt grateful.

During one of my appointments Dr. Moshman told me he was going to help me get through this, and he did. I read recently that there is a shortage of doctors going into family medicine, and I find that alarming. We need more doctors like him.

So now it was time to meet my plastic surgeon and fourth doctor, Dr. Thompson. We had our first appointment with him on June 16. This was my 20th appointment in 12 weeks and Bruce had gone with me to nearly all of them. I was beginning to feel entitled to frequent flyer miles.

While we were on the way to our first meeting with Dr. Thompson, Bruce said, "Come on, let's go pick out a new one." (He actually used a word that rhymes with "tube.") I thought he summed up the process perfectly. It's like a fun-house mirror version of picking out new kitchen cabinets, only instead of deciding between oak or maple you're deciding between silicone and saline.

Dr. Thompson asked me how much I knew about my choices and I told him I knew I could have implants or use my own tissue and I was pretty sure I wanted implants. (When it comes to surgery, I'm in the "less is more" camp.) He told me he didn't do the tissue surgery because the cosmetic results typically are not as good. And I said I knew my implant choices were silicone or saline and I was leaning toward silicone because I had read saline didn't feel as natural. I wasn't worried about rupturing or leaking or any of those Hollywood horror stories. He said the contents are like a gummy bear so leaking isn't an issue.

He actually let us hold an implant, which was helpful if a bit trippy. I felt like I was supposed to say something but wasn't sure what, so I said, "It feels boobish."

I noticed he had a silhouette of Nefertiti on his lab coat as part of his plastic surgeons' society logo and asked him if she was on there because she's pretty. He said yes, she's considered an ideal of beauty. Then he said sometimes the Venus di Milo is also used and showed me a couple of wall certificates featuring her as well.

I refrained from saying that an armless woman might not be the best role model for plastic surgery.

You can tell a guy knows what he's doing when during his first inspection of the area in question, he says, "So what are you—a (insert bra size here)?" and gets it right, before he even gets the tape measure out.

I mentioned that I didn't always remember whom I had informed of my decisions. When we went to see Dr. Kingston the following week to schedule the mastectomy, I didn't realize I hadn't told him about my decision. He asked where we go from here and I became thoroughly confused and looked over at my ombudsman and translator. Bruce explained, "You haven't told him yet." You know how conventional wisdom says take someone to appointments with you when you have a big diagnosis? Bruce is living proof this is a good idea. So I told Dr. Kingston I decided to go ahead with the mastectomy.

Bruce asked him if it would be a simple mastectomy (where only breast tissue and nipple are removed) or radical mastectomy (where pretty much everything—breast tissue, nipple, lymph nodes and muscles beneath the breast—is removed). At this point, Bruce was asking at least as many questions as I was, and I still didn't want too much detail. Some of it actually made me a bit squeamish. I mean, nipple rings gross me out and this obviously goes well beyond that. I couldn't look at surgery drawings or reconstruction pictures and couldn't read any detailed explanations. At the previous visit with Dr. Moshman, Bruce asked some very detailed questions and Dr. Moshman started to answer them until he saw my face.

When Bruce asked about the mastectomy type, Dr. Kingston explained that radical mastectomies have become pretty rare so it would be a simple mastectomy. Then he said, "I never have liked that term. Simple for whom?" and I said, "THANK you." He just so completely gets it.

I had a notebook with questions about exercise and some other things and when I said I had a few questions too, Dr. Kingston smiled and said, "I'll try to keep up." I said, "I can't even keep up," and it was true. My brain was still in hamster-wheel mode. Writing your questions down is another tenet of the cancer adventure, because it's a given that you won't remember what you wanted to ask. What's amazing is how hard it is to focus on what you want to ask even after you wrote it down. I left more than one appointment with something I forgot to ask, in spite of my notes.

Now we just had to land on a date. There's something a tad surreal about fitting a mastectomy into your schedule. I kept thinking of one my favorite cartoons from *The New Yorker*, where a guy is on the phone in his office saying, "No, Thursday's out. How about never—is never good for you?"

We settled on July 15, three weeks away. That may seem like quite a wait time, especially since I had been so impatient for some of this. But I had just hired Mary after a couple of weeks of interviews and wanted to be around for awhile before I bailed on her. She was going to start on June 30, so that gave us two weeks together.

Dr. Kingston hadn't offered an opinion on what he thought I should do, and I hadn't asked him for one. I had plenty of opinions swirling around in my head and didn't want to solicit another one. But as we were leaving that day, he put his hand on my shoulder and said I made the right decision. He said he would have been nervous if I had opted for radiation. I thought that was a really kind thing to say.

Dr. Kingston also understood that I might need something a little beyond the usual IV drugs to feel calm before the big "M." Whatever they put in your IV is actually pretty darn good—you suddenly feel this whoosh! course through your body and you feel at peace with the world. I finally understood why Bruce had a big smile on his face when they wheeled him away for his surgeries.

The only problem is, they don't give those great IV drugs to you soon enough. You still have to get from your bed to the shower to the car to the waiting room to pre-op. You have all the time in the world to fall apart. My big ambition for this surgery was to not be a crying mess when they wheeled me in. I'd done plenty of crying already and as I mentioned, I prefer doing that in private.

So during our last visit with Dr. Kingston before this mother of all surgeries, Bruce asked him if we could both take something to help us be calm for it. He said we could both take Ativan. I said, "Really? I can take it too?" and he said sure.

I had a visit coming up with Dr. Moshman for my rescheduled physical on July 1 so I figured I'd just ask him for the prescription. At this time the visits were piling up and when I came in he greeted me by saying, "So, are you seeing enough doctors lately?" and laughed. I said, "No, I think I need to see a few more."

This was the fifth time I'd seen Dr. Moshman in 12 weeks, and the first time it felt normal. We chatted about the upcoming Husker football season and other routine stuff. He was at a different office that day and his nurse Kathy was with him and I was so happy to see them both you'd think I hadn't just seen them five weeks earlier.

I noticed his knuckles were all banged up and asked him why and he said it was from cutting down trees after a big storm we had the night before. Apparently he was a tree surgeon in a former life and it came in handy now. Some hurricane-force straight line winds had come through the Omaha area and knocked out quite a few trees and damaged the roof of the Qwest Center. Bruce and I were supposed to go to an outdoor Willie Nelson concert that night with our friends Jim and Cindy but the concert was canceled because of the storm.

When I asked Dr. Moshman for the Ativan prescription, he understood why Bruce would need it but didn't initially pick up on why I would. He said, "What do you need it for? They're going to give you something," and I said, "Not soon enough," and then he understood. Even if I wasn't crying, I was afraid they might have to peel me off the ceiling or hose me off or both. I have a real attractive habit of sweating like a horse when I get super nervous. The more I thought about it, the better the Ativan sounded. I was also pretty sure I wouldn't sleep all that well the night before, and neither would Bruce. When I asked Dr. Moshman if I could start taking it two or three nights ahead of the event to help me sleep, he said yes.

I also needed to let Dr. Soori know what I decided. I had a follow-up appointment with him the next day, July 2. Like Dr. Moshman, he scheduled visits more often during the beginning. I think they do this in part to make sure you aren't stalling.

I could tell Dr. Soori was really happy I opted for the mastectomy. Oncologists don't always get happy outcomes. Sometimes they have to prepare people for the worst. Sometimes they have to watch patients make bad choices. I was one of the lucky ones; I wasn't in an immediate fight for my life. And by choosing the best possible outcome, I wasn't going to be.

I mentioned that Dr. Soori asked me to keep an open mind during our first visit. He told me that some women insist on getting a mastectomy, even though it's clear that they would do equally well with breast-conserving surgery and radiation. And he said others want to preserve their breast at all costs, even when it means a huge gamble with bad odds.

At one point while I was trying to figure out what to do, he said, "We won't let you do anything stupid." That was reassuring but also interesting because he made it clear he'd support my decision either way. So after I decided on the mastectomy, I asked him if I was being stupid and he laughed and said, "Oh no, I think you are being very smart."

Dr. Soori has more initials after his name than alphabet soup, but he wears it lightly and he's very user-friendly. He did go a bit academic on me at one point during this visit and started to say, "Now, if this were real cancer—" by which he meant invasive, and I pounced. I held my hand up and said, "It's close enough. Somebody sign me up for the fake mastectomy!"

I was comfortable with my decision and with him by then so we laughed about it. He brought "real cancer" up another time and when I started to interrupt him, he said, "I know, it's close enough!" There's an old saying, "Close only counts in horseshoes and hand grenades"—I guess we can add DCIS to that list.

This wasn't the first time I got hung up on semantics. When I was dead-set against a mastectomy, I kept calling it an amputation. Bruce kept using the "A" word after I had decided I was going to get the mastectomy and now it was like fingernails on a blackboard (or seeing a nipple ring) so I asked him to stop.

After my July 2 visit with Dr. Soori, I had nothing scheduled until the mastectomy on July 15. This was the first time I hadn't had at least one medical appointment a week since mid-March. Now there was nothing to do but wait.

The mastectomy was the new elephant in the room; I could go about my business, but it was always there. I was able to function pretty well at work and at home, but an undercurrent lay just under the surface. It wasn't the same feeling as when I was trying to decide. That truly was an emotional roller coaster, to the point where it almost felt like whiplash at times. This was more of a constant low-level hum, like a couple-three too many lattes.

I found that music helped drown out the hum, and I relied on it pretty heavily throughout this experience. You may have heard that "Music hath charms to soothe the savage breast," which sounds like a bad pun in the context of this discussion, but it just means it can help calm the noise in your head and heart.

I have liked music since I can remember. My mom bought me records (prehistoric round vinyl music delivery systems for any young people reading this) starting when I was three years old or so. The first record she ever bought me was "Wake Up Little Susie" by the Everly Brothers.

And Bruce and I are of like minds when it comes to music—

when we got married at 19, we had a waterbed (we're talking 1970s boards on the floor, not actual furniture) and his Navy footlocker. The first purchase we made as a married couple after the 1969 Pontiac Executive we paid cash for was a stereo, and we took out a loan for it. I remember Pink Floyd's "Money" was playing on the display unit and sealed the deal.

To this day, we both still listen to music a lot, but now I found myself using it nonstop to help calm that undercurrent. I was plugged in at work, at home and in transit. I'm a news junkie and my daily commutes always featured NBC or NPR, but news felt way too jarring while I was going through this.

My prescription of choice was mainly jazz standards, classical Yo-Yo Ma, Everything But The Girl, k.d. lang, Diana Krall or Bonnie Raitt, but once in awhile I got the urge to crank up something like Garbage or Santana and dance. I recommend trying it. You know how they say to dance like no one's watching? Well, no one is watching. Go for it. It's hard not to feel better after you've been dancing.

As a word geek, I found myself leaning on lyrics too. It's amazing how many everyday phrases take on the significance of stone tablets when you are dealing with a medical condition. I took great comfort from k.d. lang singing "the Godspeed of trust will settle the dust that we've been passing through," from "Trail of Broken Hearts" on her CD *Absolute Torch and Twang*. I played that CD and Bonnie Raitt's *Nick of Time* almost as obsessively as I did when they first came out.

Some of us turn to music, others to Scriptures. My sister-in-law Dawn sent me a beautiful card with the following from Isaiah 26:3: "You will keep in perfect peace him whose mind is steadfast, because he trusts in You." I was struck by the similarities to k.d. lang. We all have our ways of finding peace.

Bruce and I sort of psychically traded places for awhile around this time. When I was trying to choose between radiation and a mastectomy, Bruce told me he'd support my decision either way, but he was more scared for me than I was for myself.

After I made the decision and was calmer and stronger, he shared his fears with me, mainly that he didn't want me to die. He even wondered at one point if I shouldn't do the preventive bilateral mastectomy. He asked me to think about it and I paused for about 30 seconds and said, "I've thought about it. No." I told him I wasn't going to die and I'd rather deal with one breast at a time. I haven't regretted that decision for a moment and neither has he.

But your mind does play tricks on you. I would lie awake at night wondering what the next big WTF was going to be. I already experienced one big cosmic timing joke in my diagnosis so closely following Dad's death. I thought how classic it would be if something bad happened to Bruce right about now. I told him about my weird fears later and that if he died, I thought I would just cancel everything. He rightly pointed out how dumb that was.

Then I decided Bruce would be safe but our 16-year-old cat was going to die. She was a great source of comfort and I was afraid the cosmic timing gods might not let her be around for my recuperation. (The gods were merciful and she didn't die; she lived to be 18.) I kept thinking some other shoe would have to drop. You can see why the Ativan was a good idea.

I also had some seriously weird dreams around this time. One night I dreamed I was waiting to see Dr. Thompson's nurse Barbara, who happens to be his wife, and was wheeling around a hospital campus on a Segway to pass the time. I was wearing a hospital gown and the back was open and flapping in the breeze. Lovely. In another dream, Bruce and I were in a very crowded waiting room and they ushered us into a small private room that had a bed and dresser in it. We both lay down on the bed and pretty soon these small robots were crawling all over us to take our vital signs or something. They were kind of like the small spidery robots in the movie *Minority Report.*

Sleepless moments and weird dreams aside, we had a very nice weekend leading up to the surgery. Our friends Don and Bill were visiting from California. Don is from Nebraska and they were headed to his family reunion. We "inherited" Don and Bill from Bruce's brother Brad (try saying that out loud real fast—it's like "She sells seashells") and have stayed in touch in the 15 years since Brad's death. We hadn't seen them for about 10 years but it was easy to pick up where we left off. We met them downtown at a hotel Thursday night and lucked into some great jazz, and we went to dinner together on Sunday.

Our dinner spot was Lo Sole Mio, a neighborhood Italian place in Omaha, and Bill paid it the high compliment of saying it reminded him of the Italian restaurants in his childhood Brooklyn. I was a bit dressed up in light clothing, a natural magnet for spaghetti sauce, so I asked for one of their bibs. It was just like the paper gowns I had worn a dozen times in Dr. Kingston's office. The restaurant patrons are lucky I didn't do some Pavlov's dog thing and start disrobing in the restaurant. I probably came close enough because after a couple of glasses of wine I started getting a little loud about my medical adventure. Bruce told me some diners nearby were starting to shoot nervous glances in our direction so I toned it down.

It was nice to have Don and Bill around because it was great catching up with them again, and it was also great to hear them tell me how brave I was. I'm not sure I was all that brave—the undercurrent was still humming along—but hearing it makes you want to live up to it.

I had quite a few people tell me how brave I was, and on one level I started wondering if that's the cancer equivalent of people saying you look great "for your age" as you get older. I mean, if we're not shrieking and sobbing we must be brave, right? And in a way, I get that. I remember seeing women after I had heard they had breast cancer and thinking how normal they looked. It's just another one of those things you don't know until you have a front-row seat. The best explanation I can come up with is that things are just about always worse in your imagination. Certainly not everything—and the things that actually are worse are probably too awful to contemplate—but when it happens to you, you just deal with it. And it's only one small facet of who you are.

And although I still think my bravery was questionable, on another level I think I was getting better at living in the moment. Yes, I have big scary surgery on Tuesday—but this is Thursday, and the food, drink, jazz and friends are great. I really believe that's one of the lessons cancer can teach us.

It also helped that after two attempts at breast-conserving surgery, I had time to get used to my breast changing shape. I had started thinking of it as the Incredible Shrinking Boob. We were just going to carry this to its logical conclusion. I was able to have immediate reconstruction, so that helped too. I wouldn't be completely flat when I came out of it. I was grateful for that physical and mental head start, but I was still nervous. Like I said, this ain't no gallbladder.

The mastectomy was scheduled at a different facility from the one where I had my previous two surgeries. It's closer to where we live, smaller and more intimate, and it's where Dr. Thompson usually does his surgeries. Dr. Thompson and Dr. Moshman also have their offices in that building. I knew this would be much better for Bruce. He hated the waiting room in the other facility because it was big and crowded and most of the people in it seemed stressed out or sad.

Since I'd be spending the night, Dr. Kingston warned me that the rooms were small and I told him that didn't matter. I was just going to be conked out in bed, so what difference did it make? The rooms are private so that was a big plus. Dr. Moshman's nurse Kathy told me I'd have to request a private room if I went to the other facility and might have to wait until I could get one, which I would have done without question. I don't even sign up for a roommate when my employer has one of our out-of-town national conferences and no one is hooked up to a catheter then. I have to pay extra to get my own room and to me it's money well spent.

July 15 was the big day. We popped our Ativan like a good little boy and girl and off we went. I tried to stay focused on what we were starting, not what we were ending.

Dr. Kingston was an incredibly reassuring presence that morning. He had been funny and comforting through the previous surgeries and office visits, but he was nothing short of amazing this time.

When he came to see me in pre-op, he was wearing a blue suit and looked great. So being both drugged-up and conversationally brilliant, I said, "You look great." (I probably should give you a little context here. I took pictures of my doctors and nurses and other staff to chronicle my adventure, and responses from friends when they saw his picture ranged from Mary's "He looks like a movie star playing a doctor," to Teresa's "Wow, he's really handsome," to Audrey simply saying, "Whoa.")

He deflected my druggy compliment by saying, "I guess that's better than saying I didn't recognize you with your clothes on." I was half-flying on Ativan by then and don't remember if I laughed but I thought it was funny.

Then I must have looked scared because his expression changed and he came over and put his arm around me. There's not much you can say at a time like that, and he didn't try.

I'm not sure I can convey how powerful that simple gesture was. I wanted to put my arm around his waist but I was afraid they'd have to pry me off of him, so I patted his stomach. He noticed I had blood on my hand from the IV prep and asked the nurse for a sterile wipe. She said, "I can do that," and he said, "We're fine," and wiped the blood from my hand.

He could have said, "I've got it," or "No problem," or even,

"I'm fine." Instead, he said, "*We're* fine," and I was no longer a frightened woman alone in a curtained-off area before they let my husband join me. I was not facing this scariest of surgeries alone, and I will always be grateful to him for that moment. They don't teach that in medical school.

Nurses at the facility where I had my previous surgeries let Bruce join me right away so he was in the room while they prepped me. This facility had a different protocol. My nurse, Ann, explained that she didn't like anyone distracting her from her patients, and I can see where that makes sense if they're tense or squeamish or attention hogs. Bruce has a problem with needles so when they were hooking up my IV at the other facility, I'd ask him if he was okay. And he was fine but I liked having him to focus on. This time I had nothing to focus on but me, so Dr. Kingston was a welcome distraction.

He may have been a bit too distracting because I completely missed Ann placing the anti-nausea patch on my neck while he was there. After he left, my anesthesiologist came in and I told him I didn't think I got my patch. He started to scurry around and Ann said, "I gave you your patch, you were just too distracted by Dr. Kingston." So I said, "Sorry."

I'm sure she's seen worse, but I felt for Ann. First she had to contend with loopy, distracted me. Then Bruce and our friends Jim and Cindy showed up. You'd have to know Jim. He has a heart the size of Texas but he's capable of making some pretty borderline jokes. He asked if they were sharpening the samurai swords. Ann shot him a look that said she wouldn't mind trying one on him, but I said, "It's okay, he's here for comic relief."

When they wheeled me out to the hallway where Bruce and I would part ways, Ann told us we were under the mistletoe now. We took our cue and kissed each other before they wheeled me away. We would have in any case but that was such a nice way to put it. She's definitely been to this rodeo before.

I don't recall how long the surgery took; I'm guessing

something like two and a half hours for both procedures. First Dr. Kingston performed the mastectomy. He also removed 10 lymph nodes to be biopsied just in case cancerous cells had escaped from the breast. If they had, this is the first place they'd be likely to show up. Normally you won't have a sentinel node biopsy for DCIS, but I had so much of it my team thought it would be best to get the biopsy as a precaution.

When Dr. Kingston finished removing the tissue, Dr. Thompson inserted the expander. He also installed some engineered tissue called AlloDerm to create a better platform for the subsequent implant.

I came to several hours later in a little room and felt groggy but no big ouch pain or anything. It was too early for that. Bruce was there but Jim and Cindy weren't. He had sent them on a secret mission that I wouldn't know about for a couple of days. They showed up a little later and brought something for each of us. We had gone out with them a couple of weeks earlier and Cindy was wearing some really cute sandals that I admired. She brought me a pair of the same sandals. They also smuggled in a little cooler for Bruce so he could relax and have a cocktail while he hung out with me. It's not the easiest thing for a guy to watch his wife go through. Jim told me later that Bruce got a little tearful when they went out to eat while I was in surgery.

That was another great thing about this facility; they tell the family they can leave and then call them when it's time to come back, and they have the timing down perfect. You aren't afraid to leave the room like you were at the big facility.

Bruce asked me to watch the door while he made a drink, which was kind of like asking a sleepwalker to direct you to the library. I was pretty tuned out and every once in awhile would remember to look at the door although I'm not sure I remembered why.

Luckily, no one showed up so Bruce wasn't busted. If anyone had, we would have been better off with Dr. Kingston than one of the nurses. He gets it that patients live in the real world. When he stopped by the next morning to see how I was doing, I asked him if I could have a glass of champagne on our wedding anniversary the following day. He asked which one, wished us many more and then said, "Sure, have two if you want."

After he left the room my nurses got a bit jacked up. One said, "I never would have recommended that," and the other one said, "I just pretended I didn't hear him." I told him about that later and he laughed.

I had never spent the night in a hospital and was a bit surprised to find out you don't sleep all that well. And in this intimate facility, there was just me and my nurse Barb. It couldn't have been more peaceful. There were thunderstorms in the area so we'd hear thunder once in awhile, but even that seemed peaceful.

Barb is one of the nicer human beings on the planet. She's beautiful and kind and we chatted about all kinds of stuff. I got seriously lucky when it turned out she was also my nurse for the second-stage reconstruction three and a half months later.

She kept asking me how my pain was and I didn't have a clue. At one point I just randomly said "Four" because it sounded right for "Not horrible and not sure I can tell anyway." I don't remember if I stuck with "Four" or decided to mix it up with a "Three" here and there. I truly do not get that scale.

Barb offered to give me a sponge bath and I said no thanks so she handed me the washcloth. I was thinking to myself, "Not without a video crew and some hideous boom-chicka-boom soundtrack," but thought it would be best not to say that out loud. My friend Jim isn't the only one capable of tasteless jokes.

I found out that cell phones and iPods are two of the world's greatest inventions when you're in the hospital. I liked getting Bruce's text messages wishing me good night and good morning. And it was nice for him because when I texted back he knew it was okay to call, which he did at 4 a.m. If I recall correctly, that was about the time my catheter came out so I even had news to report ("catieter out.") My text messages looked like ransom notes, they had so many typos in them.

"Goodnight, sweetie. I love you."

"Me tno"

Having the iPod was great because middle-of-the-night TV ranges from poor to sad. I felt pretty lucky to run across the movie *M*A*S*H* until they got to a big bloody surgery scene. Oh, look, surgery—my favorite! Time for music! I learned bluegrass is a little too cranked up for 2 a.m.; jazz is much better.

They do offer sleeping pills but I was worried I'd be too groggy at discharge time so I declined. I wanted to get out of there as soon as I could and go sleep in my own bed.

Dr. Kingston came to see me bright and early as promised the next morning, greeting me with a "Hey, pal." He came over and held my hand, then took my pulse and peered at my bandage. I'm not sure what they expect to see when they do that—looks like a bandage to me. But I also had a couple of surgical drains hanging off my left side; I'm sure they were more visually interesting. Barb had shown me how to drain them, which she did a couple times during the course of the night, and she also showed Bruce.

We got my follow-up visit with Dr. Thompson set for Friday to get my surgical dressings changed. Dr. Kingston told me I was good to go and that he'd see me the following week. But I couldn't go home just yet because Dr. Moshman was also planning to stop by. It was kind of fun being in the building where he worked. It was nice to see him, and his nurse Kathy had stopped by the previous afternoon. She told me I looked great and I have nothing to compare myself to so I believed her. But now I wonder if she wasn't just being kind. I've seen pictures of myself after the stage 2 reconstruction/augmentation surgery and my eyes are so puffy and creased it looks like airbags went off under them. I thought I was scary looking.

It took Dr. Moshman awhile to get there. Probably no longer than half an hour but I was dressed and raring to get out of there so it seemed like forever. He apologized for being late and said he forgot he was going to stop by. I roughed him up a bit for forgetting about me, but it didn't faze him. He just said, "I knew you'd be fine."

Like Dr. Kingston, he came over and took my pulse and peeked at the bandage. And then he did the nicest thing. He asked me how I was, of course, and then he turned to Bruce and asked him how he was. He gets it that two of you are going through this.

I don't remember her name, I think it's Judy, but the woman who runs the short-stay unit walked me to the door (did I mention I don't like wheelchairs?) and told me I hit the Trifecta with Drs. Moshman, Kingston and Thompson. Another nurse called them "The Dream Team."

I felt that way too. I was grateful to all of them, and to Dr. Soori, for getting me this far. The toughest part of the journey was behind me. Now it was time to focus on recovery.

Chapter 4:

Surgical Drains and the Well-Dressed Woman: Recovering from Mastectomy

Whether it's breast cancer or something else, having your body call the shots is a humbling experience. My body has always done what it needed to without much complaint, and my attitude toward it ranged from benign neglect to outright abuse until I approached 50 and realized diet and exercise might not be such a bad idea (in moderation, of course). Coping with physical restrictions after my mastectomy and concurrent first-stage reconstruction was a real eye-opener.

I didn't realize this surgery was serious business until Dr. Thompson said I would need to miss two weeks of work and wouldn't be able to drive during that time. I was also going to have to sleep on my back for two weeks.

The back sleeping was going to take some getting used to since I'm a fairly devout side sleeper, not to mention my cat likes lying on my chest when I'm on my back. But as with everything else, there was a reason for it. Dr. Thompson explained that he didn't want me accidentally dislodging the teardrop-shaped tissue expander by sleeping on my side, and that it takes about two weeks for the tissue to heal enough to immobilize the expander in place.

Other instructions included no lifting more than 10 pounds with my right hand, and no lifting the left (mastectomy) arm above the shoulder. Walking was okay, but he initially wanted me babying that arm to the point where I didn't even allow it to swing when I walked. Nor did I realize I was going to have to take sponge baths for a week. This was all doable but highly annoying; especially the shower restriction because it reminded me of camping.

I was released on a Wednesday and Bruce took that day and the rest of that week off to be with me. Wednesday was pretty uneventful for the most part—at that point, I was still pretty much sleeping off the anesthetic and catching up on the sleep I didn't get on my overnight stay.

One memorable thing about that first day was the flowers and plants starting to show up. I had three deliveries that day and several more over the next couple of days. Our house started looking like a funeral home, which is not exactly the analogy I was looking for. The only conclusion I could reach is that breasts generate a lot of sympathy. My brother-in-law Jim was fighting off a recurrence of bladder cancer at the time and he joked that no one sent him flowers. And when I had my gallbladder removed the following year, I got one bouquet and was surprised to get that.

I discovered that overall, the breast cancer swag is great. Jim and Cindy had given me a diamond palm tree necklace as soon as I was diagnosed. I wore it to most of my pre-mastectomy appointments in the mistaken belief it might bring me luck. Although it didn't ward off the mastectomy, I still liked it. Audrey came over with homemade food and a basket of gifts from my friends at work. My friend Janie gave me a pretty black camisole for "the girls."

And Bruce gave me trendy reading glasses after each breast-conserving surgery. It reminded me of when I was in first grade and my mom rewarded me with a book after I got the required shots for school. In some ways, you can really make out on this breast cancer thing.

All mercenary considerations aside, it was wonderful to be reminded how much people care and it really made me appreciate my family and friends. That's practically a cancer cliché, I know. But think about it. Clichés are clichés because they're overused, right? Perhaps they're overused because they're true. We go through so much of our lives caught up in our daily routines and living in our own little worlds that we hardly notice the people we care for, and who care for us, until something like cancer happens. Finding myself surrounded by so much love and care was both humbling and uplifting.

That first day really wasn't bad on the recovery front. I was more tired than anything and very glad to recover at home. I'd learned from my first two surgeries that anesthesia alone made me feel pretty tired and stupid.

The only thing I missed about the hospital was the bed, which I realized the first time I tried to sit up. Hospital beds are great because you don't have to use any of your own muscles to get to a sitting position. You push a button and the bed does all the work.

I had no idea that having a mastectomy would have any impact on sitting up. After all, your breasts don't actually do anything except hang off of your body. But Dr. Thompson had to cut into the chest wall to place the tissue expander that served as my temporary implant, so when I sat up, my wounded chest wall complained. It wasn't as bad as the sudden, searing Pow! of the stereotactic biopsy, but it was close enough to make me realize I actually had some pretty significant surgery.

As I mentioned, I had doctor's orders to sleep on my back for two weeks, and I was afraid of accidentally rolling over on my side so I slept in our reclining chair the first night. Bruce slept on the sofa next to me to keep me company.

I hated sleeping in that recliner. I woke up once in the middle of the night and could not get the chair to an upright position. I felt like a turtle that had been flipped over on its back and I did not like that powerless feeling one bit. After that first night, I just piled pillows up next to me in bed to prevent rolling over and it worked pretty well.

The worst pain was the first three or four days, and it wasn't constant, mainly when I was trying to get from lying down to sitting up. You may not be able to do this without help; one of my friends told me she couldn't. I was usually able to manage. I could swing around to get my legs over the bed and hoist myself up from my right side. Bruce was more than willing to help and if he was around and awake I let him. He wanted me to wake him up if he was sleeping but I refused to do that. For me, asking for help is an 8 on that famous pain scale, even from my roommate of 30-plus years.

Two days after the mastectomy, we celebrated our 33rd wedding anniversary. I was drugged up, banged up, taped up and able to do nothing much in the way of celebrating but it was one of the nicest anniversaries we've ever had. I think it even outweighs our wedding day. That always will be a wonderful memory and milestone but this was infinitely sweeter. On the day you get married, you don't really have a clue. Going through something like this together makes marriage worth the price of admission.

Bruce pulled the anniversary surprise of our lives that day. He's done it to me more than once and I always fall for it. He asks me to get something out of a kitchen cabinet or the glove box on our way to dinner and there's the little box from Borsheims, which is the Omaha version of Tiffany & Co. You see that silver box with the burgundy ribbon and you know you're in for something good.

We were having champagne and chocolate in bed and he handed me the telltale silver box. I opened it and saw a diamond on a chain. I made some comment about how pretty it was and he said, "That's your wedding ring." I wasn't exactly a brain trust on the pain pills and champagne so I said, "No, it's not, it's a necklace."

Then he handed me a ring box, which was my wedding set with a new and considerably larger diamond. If I hadn't been so out of it, I would have cried but I was lucky just to keep up with the plot. The necklace was the original diamond from my engagement ring, which he gave me when we were both 18.

Remember I mentioned Bruce had sent our friends Jim and Cindy on a secret mission while I was in the hospital? It turns out the mission was to send them to Borsheims to upgrade my ring, which he had smuggled out. The woman helping them placed a rush order on it to make sure it was ready in time for our anniversary two days later. Bruce even had the ring box hiding in plain sight in my nightstand drawer to pique my curiosity, but I just thought it was an empty box I had forgotten about. Of course, my stunning new bling paled in comparison to the grilling book I gave him.

I know how spoiled I am and not just on the jewelry front. Major illness brings out the best or worst in people. I've read about and heard about husbands and boyfriends who just can't deal with breast cancer, to the point where some of them even leave, but it brought out the best in my husband. He was and continues to be my best friend—luckily, he's a friend with benefits.

Among all the flowers that showed up, Jim and Cindy sent us a bouquet of 33 roses to celebrate our 33 years. A couple of family members also focused on our anniversary instead of my surgery and I really liked that. Although make no mistake, flowers for whatever reason are more than welcome.

I mentioned to Bruce at one point that day that I felt great and he laughed and said, "No wonder, you're on pain pills and champagne." And it *was* great—I didn't feel a thing! It was probably the best I felt for a couple of weeks.

Speaking of pain pills, I took my last pain pill on Friday morning, three days after surgery. I switched to extra strength Tylenol because I didn't like the floaty feeling I got from the Roxicet, except when I mixed it with champagne. (I know, I know, bad patient—I can just see my short-stay nurses covering their eyes.) Not to mention no fewer than six people told me they'd make me constipated, starting with Dr. Kingston when he visited me in the hospital. By the time my brother-in-law Jeff, a former medic, told me, I felt like Ralphie in *A Christmas Story*.

We had our first follow-up with Dr. Thompson that Friday. I'd been going commando, so to speak, until that moment, but now it was time to get me into a stretchy surgical bra, which was going to be my new best friend for awhile since Dr. Thompson wanted me wearing it day and night. He explained later that the bra prevented the weight of the partially filled tissue expander from placing excessive pressure on the thin chest tissue and eroding it.

Maneuvering me into the bra took a bit of doing, given the drains and my inability to raise my arm. Barbara said, "How many people does it take to put on a surgical bra?" while both of them were trying to wrestle me into it. Apparently three.

I came home with a fair amount of tape residue on my torso from the dressings. They sent some adhesive remover along and said I could probably get more from the hospital pharmacy, but I didn't check. (I did check Walgreen's and they do not carry it.) I heard that rubbing alcohol, baby oil or nail polish remover also work. I had the best luck with rubbing alcohol but immediately washed afterward since it's so drying. I had some luck with baby oil and no luck at all with nail polish remover. Whichever one you try, don't use it near an incision.

One of the most annoying aspects of recovery was the surgical drains. My doctors each had a different nickname for them. Dr. Kingston called them my friends; Dr. Thompson called them suitcases. Dr. Moshman's preferred term was hand grenades, which they actually resemble. They're small plastic bulbs attached to your body by thin tubes inserted under your skin near your incision and held in place by a suture, and you need to empty them regularly and swab antibiotic ointment on the area where they connect to your body after you shower (once you can start showering). I had two of them; one for the breast area and one for the lymph node area.

We had to empty them about four times a day to start with but that gradually slowed down, and we had to pour the liquid into a little measuring cup and record how much liquid we were getting from each drain. The recording sheet had room for up to four drains. I couldn't figure out why anyone would need four drains until I realized some women get both breasts done at once. Two of them were such a nuisance I can't even imagine what having four of them hanging off your body would be like.

We had to take the drainage log sheet along to appointments so Dr. Thompson could see how it was progressing, like the surgical version of a report card. He said he usually waits until fluid output is less than one ounce in 24 hours before removing the drains, because at this level the body can reabsorb the fluid without it accumulating around the implant.

I keep saying "we," but I never once had to manage the drain process. Bruce helped me in the beginning when I couldn't manage it myself but then he just kept doing it and it turned into our little ritual. He "milked" the liquid the length of the tube, from the entry point to the drainage bulb, then emptied the contents into the measuring cup and measured the results.

He washed his hands and put on latex gloves every time like Barb showed him. One day he decided to do drain duty right before he got in the shower so he got undressed. The sight of my six-foot-tall husband clad only in latex gloves cracked me up for some reason, which got him started, and then neither one of us could stop laughing. Bruce Fox, Male Nurse. Quick, somebody cue up the bad soundtrack!

The drains are somewhat visually startling at first because the contents are kind of a tomato-juice red, but the liquid eventually looks more like pale tea. Showering with them isn't that tough but it's a nuisance having to haul them around and attach them to your clothes. I usually pinned them to my bra or the underside of my shirt. You can pin them to your slacks but you want to be careful not to forget about them and accidentally yank on them if you're changing clothes or going to the bathroom. I accidentally had my hand on one as I was getting out of bed one morning, so when I pushed off I gave it a good tug. That wasn't particularly pleasant.

A lot of the general discomfort you feel, such as when bending over, is from the drains. I had no idea drains were causing this discomfort until Dr. Thompson's other nurse, Robyn, explained it to me.

I was able to get rid of the lymph node drain after a week, but had to keep the second one for three weeks. I was a bit bummed when I found out I had to keep it that long. Robyn explained you need them for a longer time if they use AlloDerm to help build a platform for the implant, like they did for me. I still didn't understand the difference so I asked Dr. Thompson. He explained that having both an expander and artificial dermis present prompts an inflammatory reaction.

It was kind of funny when they removed the first drain because Bruce was with me, as he had been for at least two dozen appointments, and he realized he probably didn't want to stay in the room for this particular event. Robyn said, "Good, I don't want to have to pick anyone up off the floor today."

When Dr. Thompson pulled the drain tubing out he said, "Take a deep breath." So I did, and he yanked, and I felt it. And boy, did that area feel less sore after it was out. Sometimes you don't realize how sore you are until you aren't anymore.

One of my less stellar moments involved clothes shopping while still sporting the second drain. Dr. Thompson had just cleared me to drive so I went to this appointment by myself and found out I would be stuck with the drain for another week. I decided I needed "drain-appropriate" (baggy) clothing for work, so I left Dr. Thompson's office and headed to the department store. It was a thrill to be driving, although I found out I had to be careful twisting around and pushing the door or I'd feel it.

I still had a limited range of motion and it did not occur to me that this might cause problems trying on clothes. I was aware enough to try to find things that button or zip, but the only items available that weren't too fitted were pajamas or exercise wear. So I cluelessly grabbed a handful of pullover tops, and the second one I tried on got stuck halfway over my head with my drain hanging out.

I had nightmare visions of what would happen next.

First Sales Clerk: "What are those retching noises coming from the dressing rooms?"

Second Sales Clerk: "Beats me, but Courtney just went back there to help a customer; maybe she knows."

I finally yanked my arm into an overhead position and escaped the shirt. I left the store with some new clothes and a throbbing armpit.

The shopping fiasco was a couple of days before I went back to work. I'm very lucky to work at a place that offers short-term disability and let me work part-time for two weeks after I got back from my two-week break. I felt kind of sheepish about doing that, but Audrey told me she had done it after hers and was glad she did. Like me, she felt a little embarrassed about taking that time and like her, I'm glad I did it. I didn't realize how hard it can be just to sit at a computer.

I was really uncomfortable and tired the first couple of days after I went to work, and I'd go home and take naps of a couple-three hours, but it gradually got better. Mary, my office roommate, told me I was walking a little funny the first few days. Bruce also noticed that I had my left shoulder hiked up. I didn't even notice I was doing it and was afraid it might stay that way, like when your mom tells you your face will freeze into whatever disobedient expression you happen to have on it. Luckily it didn't.

A couple of weeks after surgery, I started noticing my armpit and triceps were numb, along with burning sensations I hadn't felt before. Dr. Kingston explained the burning was nerve ends and that it was temporary. And he was right, those sensations subsided after a few days. It was weird to think of my body following a timeline for something like that. It was a perfectly logical trajectory as far as my brain and nerves and skin were concerned but just one more mystery to me.

Numbness is a different story. The numbness in my triceps evaporated but I can't say the same thing for my armpit. It may or may not go away completely, depending on how many lymph nodes were removed, because as Dr. Kingston explained it, skin nerves traversing the area have been affected. A friend of mine had 17 lymph nodes removed and her armpit is still numb two years later. Mine (a year and a half later, after removing 10) has subsided for the most part, but it hasn't gone away completely. Dr. Kingston said that happens a lot; you just get used to it.

Shaving a numb armpit was an adventure. I have to admit I didn't worry about it too much the first couple of weeks, which wasn't like me B.C. (Before Cancer). I typically don't wear makeup and I spend about two minutes a day on my hair, but I'm not relaxed to the extent of parading my leg or armpit hair. But at this point I was no longer worried about making an impression on my doctors and nurses. I figure they've seen it all before and one more hairy armpit wouldn't faze them. (Now that I've been around them handling various body parts and fluids, I don't have a clue what *would* faze them and I'm sure I don't want to know.)

Bruce shaved it for me the first time because I was afraid to. I switched to an electric razor for awhile to avoid shredding my armpit with a manual razor. It also had a hollow spot caused by removing the lymph nodes that I couldn't quite get to so I called it my soul patch. I've become acclimated so I can shave it now with a regular razor, although the divot is still there.

Three weeks after surgery, I was finally able to get rid of that second drain. I kept thinking this one had more time to get itself entrenched so I was prepared for it to be more painful than removing the first one. Dr. Thompson and I were chatting about something or other as he was preparing the area and I asked him when he was going to take it out. He said, "It's out," and I said, "You're kidding." What a relief! It sure felt good to get rid of those drains.

I know I've gone on at some length about drains but it just felt weird to be going about my daily routine with this foreign thing hanging from my body. I felt a bit like a science experiment and also like I was walking around with this gross medical secret. I wondered how many other people were going around with surgical drains and newly minted scars and other medical accoutrements the rest of us couldn't see.

The Willie Nelson concert that had been canceled because of the storm was rescheduled for roughly a week after my surgery, when I was still packing a drain. We went and I was fine, but Bruce was like a fidgety Secret Service agent. He was blocking and tackling to make sure no one bumped into me.

And it briefly occurred to me that I should have tried to capitalize on my status, like wearing a big pink "Survivor" T-shirt and marching up to the front of the stage; in hopes of what, I don't know. A bandana? An invitation to get high on his bus? I'm not sorry I kept a low profile but I am sorry I forgot to take my camera. He was really good about letting people come right up to the stage and take his picture.

During the concert, Bruce gave me the type of compliment only a husband can give. Willie was singing a song about how "I'll have to get over you again," and Bruce leaned over and said, "That would be a great song at your funeral."

I replied, "Don't rush me."

One week after getting rid of the last drain, and four weeks after surgery, I started working on my range of motion. I was a bit worried because my armpit was pretty locked up, with a general feeling of tightness replacing the burning sensation. I hoped I wouldn't need physical therapy, and I didn't; the exercises Dr. Kingston gave me worked.

Some of the exercises took longer than others, but my full range of motion was restored within three weeks. The classic one, the one everyone who's been through it tells you about, is the "wall crawl." It has two variations. In one, you stand facing the wall and you crawl your fingers up the wall as high as your arm will go. In the other one, you do the same thing but you're perpendicular to the wall. You do the crawl with both arms and in the beginning, you certainly can tell a difference in your range of motion.

The one I had the most trouble with was where you lie on the floor with your fingers laced together behind your head and your elbows next to your ears. Your goal is to bring your elbows to the floor. Piece of cake, right? But I couldn't get that left elbow within four or five inches of the floor for quite awhile.

I want to make a point here about communicating with multiple doctors, because we had a little communication glitch over the range of motion exercises. I said earlier that I didn't always remember what I said to whom as I was trying to figure out which treatment route to take. The same thing happened here. Dr. Kingston gave me the exercises but told me he was deferring to Dr. Thompson, because recovering from reconstructive surgery has a different set of requirements.

I don't remember sharing that particular bit of information with Dr. Thompson, who likely assumed I was getting instruction from Dr. Kingston. I recall asking Dr. Thompson about regular exercise such as riding a bike, but don't recall discussing range of motion exercises. I was under the impression I couldn't start those exercises until that last drain had been out for a week and just operated on that theory instead of asking him. He told me later that he wouldn't have had me wait that long.

This is where communicating gets tricky—it's easy to ask questions when you know you aren't following along. When you think you know what's going on, it still doesn't hurt to double check. So the moral of that story is to ask your doctors who's going to clear you for exercise if you're working with more than one, and let Dr. A. know what you discussed with Dr. B.

Speaking of regular exercise, Dr. Thompson cleared me to do things like ride our tandem bicycle six weeks after surgery. (He okayed sex a week or two before that though. He must figure we spend more time on the bike.)

Losing some of your independence isn't the most fun a person can have, but it could be a lot worse. Recovery is nature's way of telling you to relax. And your body needs it—I napped a lot. One of my favorite quotes from Dana Jennings, a brilliant writer who blogs about his experience with prostate cancer for *The New York Times*, was when he said he slept so much he thought he was turning into a cat.

Bruce and I have lived with cats for more than 30 years, so I can testify to their epic napping abilities. Our current feline roommate was really happy to have a companion for her snoozes. She also turned out to be surprisingly good about staying off of my chest.

When I wasn't sleeping I watched movies or read the paper or just listened to birds on the porch. I learned to scale back my expectations even regarding these enforced leisure activities. I thought I was going to get caught up on some of the books I've been meaning to read but I just didn't feel like it. And I had grand designs of watching all the subtitled movies Bruce doesn't have patience for, but they felt too much like homework. I got caught up on episodes of *The Office* and watched movies like *Ratatouille* instead. And I happened to stumble into a Peter Sellers marathon one day—sheer bliss.

Walking to the mailbox a block away became my big daily event. I dutifully kept my left hand in my pocket so I wouldn't accidentally swing my arm.

Three days after the mastectomy, Dr. Moshman called to let us know that all 10 of the lymph nodes were clear; no cancerous cells had escaped. This was great news because it meant I was finished with treatment and would only need to complete my reconstruction. I would not need to consider chemotherapy. However, the breast tissue they removed was still harboring some residual ductal carcinoma in situ cells. As Dr. Soori had said, my decision to get a mastectomy was a smart one.

While I was recovering, it took some effort to get over the

feeling that I should be doing something productive, but it's good to be reminded that you don't always have to be "doing"— sometimes it's okay to just "be." If that's a lesson cancer has to teach us, I'll take it.

But I think my biggest, most enduring lesson came five days after my surgery. I was reading the Sunday paper and while I'm not in the habit of reading obituaries to see whom I know (yet), a face jumped out at me. She was young, blond and beautiful, and she had died at age 40 of breast cancer. I thought, "God rest her soul," and then realized how incredibly lucky I am.

In the end, something is going to take me out. It just won't be breast cancer.

Chapter 5:

My $83,000 Remodeling Project

The next step in my medical adventure was getting the mastectomized breast in shape for my implant. Working with the plastic surgeon is fun because the tough part is over and you're like your own remodeling project. Demolition and site preparation are out of the way and now construction can begin.

Six weeks after surgery, I was healed enough for Dr. Thompson to start filling my temporary expander with saline. This would allow my skin to stretch enough to support the regular implant that I would receive during second-stage reconstruction.

As I mentioned, he also cleared me to start engaging in regular exercise such as riding a bike. Bruce thought this whole exercise discussion was funny. He said the way I kept asking my doctors about exercise they'd get the impression I'm really into it. I assured him they could tell by looking at me that I'm not.

I ended up getting two saline injections of 100cc each, spaced three weeks apart. This was a bit of a *Where's Waldo* experience because they use a little magnet to find the metal port in the expander where they inject the saline. It's in a small contraption similar to the one holding those perpetual motion balls on strings that were popular office toys for awhile. Dr. Thompson waved the magnet over the area until it reacted.

The saline injections were painless. I never thought to ask whether there's much leak potential, but it stayed as full as it's intended to so I imagine that's minimal. I could see the difference after each one. I felt like a bicycle tire getting pumped up.

I had an ID card showing a picture of the expander and its metal port. I was advised to have it on hand at airports. It even had a little blurb on it about how the metal might set off airport detectors. I had business meetings in Tampa in September and Montreal in October so I made sure to have the card handy. I didn't set off any airport alarms, thank goodness, although I did get pulled aside for an extra bag search and questioning as I was leaving Canada.

My medical schedule up to now had still been pretty full. After the mastectomy and first-stage reconstruction on July 15, I had eight appointments and a lab visit before my first saline fill on August 26. (On July 22, I had back-to-back appointments with Dr. Kingston and Dr. Thompson, at 1:45 p.m. and 3:00 p.m. I felt like I should show up somewhere at 4 o'clock just on principle.)

But now the appointments were starting to wind down. I had my last appointment with Dr. Kingston on August 12. When I saw Dr. Soori on September 30, two months after the previous visit when he started me on Tamoxifen, he told me I didn't need to come back for three months.

I got off to a bit of a wrong start on the Tamoxifen regimen. I'm taking it daily for five years to prevent cancer from showing up in the other breast. Because it increases the risk for blood clots, Dr. Soori prescribed a daily low-dose aspirin. I mistakenly bought regular dose aspirin so I was taking 325 mg a day instead of 81 mg. I sprouted some massive dark purple bruises on my legs until I started taking the right dosage. You might want to pay closer attention than I did.

I scheduled the second-stage reconstruction for December 1. This procedure would also include getting an implant for the other breast ("augmentation") and lifting it ("mastopexy") so they would match better. That may not even be an issue for you, but it was for me. I'll try not to be too graphic but there was zero symmetry after the first-stage reconstruction. One resembled a bowling ball and the other one a bowling pin. Gravity is not pretty.

I could have scheduled it sooner but I didn't have the sense of urgency I felt when I was trying to figure out what to do. I didn't want to go through surgery and recovery during Husker football season, and we had planned a vacation in Cabo San Lucas, Mexico, during the middle of November. I finally felt like I was putting cancer on my schedule instead of the other way around.

The toughest part of my cancer journey was behind me. But I knew I had another round of surgery and recovery facing me, and taking an actual vacation was just what the doctor ordered, if you'll forgive the pun. It would be nice if everyone could take a time-out and just go somewhere when you're in the middle of something like this. It was one big "Aaahh" from the time we got there until the time we left.

I forgot about everything and I do mean everything. I didn't think about work, or surgery, or cancer. (And although my cancer is officially cured thanks to the mastectomy, I'm a marked woman. An oncology nurse told me that once you've had cancer, you're susceptible to more cancer. So now I have a standing date twice a year with Dr. Soori, in addition to an annual chest X-ray, possibly the occasional MRI, and regular blood tests. So while I don't dwell on it, I can't deny I'm living within its shadow.)

Cabo was so good at inducing forgetfulness that I actually forgot I didn't live in a warm climate. It happened during our obligatory Harley tourist shopping. Lord knows if there's one thing I don't need it's another Harley T-shirt, but I decided to make an exception for lovely Cabo. It has just a tad more panache than my hometown shirt from Minot, N.D.

Their T-shirt selection wasn't huge. The only thing I liked at all was a rather heavy long-sleeved black shirt, and I caught myself thinking, "Well, I can't wear that." It took a couple of seconds before I realized how completely I bought into the Cabo fantasy. Who was I kidding? I could wear it in three days, when I returned to cold Omaha and reality. I think a vacation is doing its job pretty well if it can make you that forgetful.

I also had a wonderful coincidence happen while I was there. G.K. Chesterton said that coincidences are spiritual puns, and based on this I'm inclined to agree with him. It definitely felt spiritual.

We went to a wonderful Italian restaurant in the marina, which is lined with restaurants and shops. This was the kind of restaurant that's so architecturally hip it takes 10 minutes to figure out how the faucet works in the ladies' room. It looked like a sewing needle and I finally figured out to push it to one side to get water. But that bathroom sure was gorgeous. I tried to take a picture but the other thing it had going on was some dead-serious mood lighting. You practically needed a flashlight. So my photographic world tour of bathrooms was not to be.

But I digress. Daline Jones, a jazz singer from California, was performing for her CD launch party so we lucked out on that score alone. Our table was near the stage and we were having a great time enjoying the beautiful weather, good food and great jazz.

After doing a few songs, she talked about how a poem that her dad wrote inspired her next song. Then she started reciting a poem I had loved in high school and forgotten about for more than 30 years. Her dad, Ted Joans, was a Beat poet, and the poem and song are called "Truth." I found myself reciting some of the long-forgotten lines with her. When she got to the end of the poem ("You have nothing to fear from the poet but the truth,") I clapped like you would for a jazz solo. Since poetry isn't quite up there with music for much of the world, I was the only one clapping. She turned to me and bowed, and I bowed back. I felt as high as if I were parasailing.

I had only recently started writing poetry again, after an absence of nearly 20 years. I wrote a couple of poems the weekend before we left and it was a real rush. Hearing her recite a poem that had meant so much to me, that her dad happened to write, felt like a sign. It was definitely a blessing and lent a touch of magic to an already wonderful and peaceful vacation.

But vacations end, as they must. December 1 rolled around and we went to the same facility where they did the mastectomy. It was like old home week. Ann wasn't taking care of me in pre-op this time, but she stopped by to say hello and so did a couple other nurses.

Even though things were much calmer on the emotional front, surgery still requires a bit of a leap of faith, and I was impressed again at how well the medical team can put you at ease. When Dr. Thompson stopped by pre-op, he said they'd have me ready for a bikini in no time, which was awfully sweet of him. I told him not without a lot more work. I was thinking I might have missed the boat by not opting for tissue replacement surgery—do they take it from your stomach?—but it wouldn't have been nearly enough.

This time one of my nurses was named Doug so it was a real coed experience. My nurse anesthetist's name was Jeff and I liked the way he told me he was going to give me a happy hour. And I was pretty happy by the time they wheeled me into surgery. Before they got to work Dr. Thompson took some "before" pictures and marked my chest area up with a blue pen. I glanced down and commented that it looked tribal and that's all I remember until I woke up in my little room.

Before I ever had surgery, I was always afraid of anesthesia because I was afraid of not waking up again. And there are risks with general anesthesia, but people go through it every day. I think my fear was partly a vestigial hangover from the prayer we all heard as kids. I think adults underestimate just how scary "Now I Lay Me Down to Sleep" can be. "Hey, wait a minute! What do you mean 'If I should die before I wake?'" I never did like that prayer; I much preferred the guardian angel one.

I think I'm well over that hump. Now I'm just in awe of how well they are able to calibrate anesthesia for the exact amount of time it takes to get you situated. I never spent time lying on that table waiting to conk out, and conversely, I never passed out before it was time to get into position. I mentioned earlier that the closest I came was seeing them bring the oxygen mask to my face, and that only happened once.

I spent the night at the short stay unit again, and I was really happy to find out Barb was my overnight nurse again. I was also happy to find out I only had one drain this time. I had feared I'd have one on each side, but the augmented breast didn't need one. And—the happy news just kept piling up—no catheter! It was like an early Christmas present.

Like my overnight stay in July, I was Barb's only patient and it was just as nice. We talked about our families and what kinds of music we like as well as medical stuff. She kept asking me if I needed anything and at one point she asked if she should sing or something because I wasn't giving her anything to do.

Although I was hooked up to an IV, I felt pretty mobile (not to mention less gross) without a catheter. So when I wanted to go to the bathroom I thought I'd get up and get squared away before calling Barb. I knew I wouldn't try leaving the room because my IV was hooked up to the wall or something. But she heard me and put on her mom voice and said, "Do I hear you moving around in there?" and I felt mildly chastened. I said something like, "Well yeah, but I wasn't going to leave."

She told me I was very independent and it's true. I'd rather walk than be pushed in a wheelchair and I'd rather go to the bathroom without an escort. I figure this is all good practice for the nursing home. Something I'm not particularly looking forward to, but the way I see it is if I end up in a nursing home that means I didn't have to die young, and if I die young (well, I guess I should amend that to "youngish,") then I didn't have to end up in a nursing home.

Text messaging was a real blessing again. Bruce and I texted each other and I also got quite a conversation going with his brother Jeff, some of it centered on some off-color humor from an HBO comedy series that's probably best not to repeat.

I also had a stuffed dog with a Husker logo T-shirt to keep me company. Bruce made it for me at the Build-A-Bear Workshop at a nearby mall while I was in surgery. He was the only guy there and said it was definitely an experience.

I should comment on that overnight stay with regard to insurance. My overnight stay after the mastectomy was mandatory. This time I was told it was optional but my insurance would pay for it. I took that as a pretty strong hint. I figure any time insurance volunteers to pay for something it must be a good thing.

The next morning we went upstairs to Dr. Thompson's office after he released me so they could check my bandages and drain, then home to log more nap time with the cat.

Recovery after this surgery was similar to the first one but there wasn't as much pain because Dr. Thompson didn't have to cut into the chest muscle this time. I was able to get rid of my only drain after three days and shower on the fourth. This was huge. He cleared me for all activity (except sitting in a hot tub) after two weeks. I had to sleep on my back again for two weeks as well, but I was getting used to it.

There was none of the burning or numbness associated with lymph node removal during the earlier surgery. I did have occasional twinges of pain in both breasts, but nothing awful or constant.

The most time-consuming requirement was to wear a really tight sports bra day and night for three months. Dr. Thompson explained the pressure helps prevent scar tissue from forming around the implants. He advised me to go a size smaller than I would normally wear if I could stand it. So I tried to do that during the day and wear my regular size at night.

I missed two weeks of work again as he recommended but I didn't need to go part time when I got back. I was tired and I took a lot of naps after work but it was getting close to Christmas and a short holiday schedule, which helped a lot.

Bruce and I weren't going anywhere for Christmas so we decided to get a couples' massage on Christmas Eve. (His idea, by the way.) Neither of us had ever had one. It was one of the most relaxing experiences I've ever had and it made me wish I had been smart enough to schedule at least one while I was on the decision roller coaster. If it's your turn on the roller coaster I encourage you to try it. If I ever end up on another cancer adventure one of the first things I'm going to do is schedule a massage. It's certainly cheaper than a trip to Mexico.

When 2009 began, I had two breast-conserving surgeries, a mastectomy, first– and second–stage reconstruction and augmentation behind me. Now all I was missing was a nipple.

After a mastectomy, the reconstructed breast has a nice shape but it's a blank slate. The final step is recreating the nipple area so your breast looks as natural as possible, first with surgery to create the nipple and then tattooing to give it color and recreate the areola (the colored area around the nipple).

Dr. Thompson told me he works with a nurse who is pretty good at tattooing. He said some of the tattoo parlors also get good results, but I told him that's a bit too reminiscent of the big motorcycle rally in Sturgis. It might be worth it just for the experience but I wasn't sure I was up for it; I might feel like I need a Harley tattoo. He agreed and said I might leave with a rose. It was fun to learn Dr. Thompson is hip to the Harley visual vernacular. Skulls are big for guys and roses are big for girls.

Nipple reconstruction was one more way this adventure reminded me of remodeling your house. If deciding on an implant was like picking out kitchen cabinets, this was like finding the right spot on the wall for a picture. Dr. Thompson advised me to put a small round Band Aid on the spot and to try different placements to see what I liked. I told him I would but would rather have his judgment. He said some women were very particular about it. It's not that I'm not, I just figure he has a much more practiced eye.

I was healed enough for us to schedule the nipple reconstruction for January 26. This really was outpatient surgery in that I was able to go home that same day. Barbara had advised me to take the rest of that day off, so Bruce and I went out to breakfast afterward.

This surgery also was truly outpatient in that it only required a local anesthetic. It was great to be able to walk into the OR under my own steam and get onto that skinny table without wondering if I'd pass out and roll off.

When surgery got under way they had me draped so I couldn't tell what was going on but I happened to glance up at one of the overhead lights and could see what Dr. Thompson was doing in its reflection. When I said, "Wow, I can see what you're doing," Beth, the nurse who was stationed behind my head, got a bit alarmed and said, "Oh, we'll move the light." I said, "I can just close my eyes." The last thing I wanted to do was mess up that man's ability to see.

But I didn't want to close my eyes—it was too interesting. If you had asked me five years ago if I would ever watch myself having surgery, I would have laughed or yakked on your shoes. I'm far from tough but I guess that's what going through five surgeries in six months will do for a person.

And I'm really glad I was awake for it because it was fascinating. Dr. Thompson created what he called a star flap, and I could see the star take shape. And then I saw a most reasonable facsimile of a nipple emerge after he sewed the flap together to create a bump.

Dr. Thompson was true to his word and it didn't hurt. I felt tugging while he was pulling the suture silk through, but that's all. The whole procedure took about 45 minutes. I couldn't resist being a smart aleck when he was done and said, "I think you need to move it a little more to the left," and everybody laughed.

New nipples have care requirements of their own, the main one being to wear an eye patch with a little hole cut in the center for roughly four weeks. The thick oval gauze pad cushions the nipple on all sides. Dr. Thompson told me the nipple would deflate a bit, and it did. I had asked him earlier if I would always look like I was in the cold food aisle, for lack of a better term. He said I wouldn't, and I don't. But it does give you a much more normal look.

About eight weeks later it was time to schedule getting the color tattooed in. I decided to see the nurse Dr. Thompson recommended. Her office is right across the street from mine and I scheduled the tattooing session for April 11 over my lunch hour.

When I got to work that morning I was shocked by the emotions that started bubbling up out of nowhere. I kept finding myself on the verge of tears. I knew I had to get out of there so I decided on the fly to take the rest of the day off after finishing my tattoo session.

I could not believe this was happening. I had read that you can get emotional as things start to wind down, but I thought I had crossed that hurdle. The only one I had said goodbye to so far was Dr. Kingston. I expected that to be hard, and it was. It's not easy to say goodbye to someone who's helped guide you through something as difficult as breast cancer, especially after three surgeries and at least a dozen office visits.

But the flood of emotion washing over me at this juncture blindsided me. I wasn't saying goodbye to anyone else—I'd still be following up with Drs. Moshman, Soori and Thompson, just not as often. The surgeries were behind me and I hadn't felt any letdown after my final one. This was just getting some color tattooed in, for crying out loud.

But there it was. I asked Audrey if that was normal and she assured me it was. She told me how on the day of her last chemotherapy treatment, a happy milestone in anyone's book, she went to lunch with her parents and started crying.

The tattoo experience itself was fine. I opted to forego the local anesthetic because I figured my breast was numb enough I wouldn't need it. And I was right. I felt a couple minor stings here and there but for the most part it was only pressure.

Another weird remodeling experience to add to my collection—

first she swabbed the area with a couple of different colors, like picking out paint for a wall, to see what matched the other side best. Then she pulled out something that looked like a wide ruler with holes of varying sizes, to size the fake areola.

Getting the color inked in dispelled every myth I ever had about getting a tattoo. I thought all people had to do was get drunk and show up, which is probably still true in Sturgis. I was back to sponge baths for five days, no strenuous exercise or hot tubbing, and I had to keep the tattoo gooped up with special ointment and secure it with Saran wrap and a gauze pad. My nurse, Dottie, explained that your body treats the color as a foreign object and wants to push it out, and the Saran wrap helps keep it in.

She said it would lose 25-30 percent of its color, which it did, and I might need to come back for a touch-up, which I did, a month later. I asked Dr. Thompson and his eagle eye for a second opinion and he agreed I should get it touched up. They're a pretty good match now.

I've heard some women skip the nipple reconstruction step, and talked to one friend who did, and I don't understand why because the surgery and tattooing are a piece of cake compared to the rest of it. I think you'd look kind of unfinished—but to each her own. There is no right or wrong way to do this.

Another reason this reminds me of remodeling your house is that everything else starts to look shabby in comparison. You know how when you remodel the family room you notice the bathroom looks completely outdated? Dr. Thompson is absolutely stellar when it comes to reversing gravity's effects, but now that I have this great perky chest I really should do something about that muffin top. And exactly when did this turkey wattle decide to show up on my neck?

On a more practical note, you should know that the augmentation implant makes mammograms more complicated, so make sure your technicians have experience with implants. The good news is that insurance pays for augmentation when it's related to breast cancer, thanks to the Women's Health and Cancer Rights Act of 1998. More good news—you no longer need a mammogram on the mastectomy side.

You should also know there are some temporary Frankenboob aspects. For me, the appearance of the augmented one took a bit of getting used to. I had gotten used to the mastectomy one shrinking and expanding, kind of like the phases of the moon.

But the first time I saw the augmented one, with its areola outlined in red, and red scars creating an upside down "T" from the areola to the bra line and along the bra line, it was startling. (That bra line scar takes the longest to heal by the way, simply because it's going to be irritated by the bra. That stayed a bit sore longer than anything else but it's healed quite well a year out, and the part of the mastectomy scar running from my new fake areola toward the middle of my chest has practically melted away.)

A couple of other items might be worth mentioning in terms of the way the implants look and feel. I mentioned silicone vs. saline implants earlier, and having had the saline in my temporary expander I can tell you that the silicone implant does feel more natural. When it was full of saline it felt kind of like a softball.

The other thing about the reconstructed breast is that it sometimes feels cool to the touch, which makes sense when you think about it. The implant isn't going to retain heat as well as natural tissue. I never noticed a reference to this phenomenon in any of the books or online venues, and it sure didn't occur to me to ask about it.

It wouldn't have been a deal breaker for me in any case. As I mentioned before, I landed pretty quickly on implants as my preferred solution. I just thought it might be worth passing along.

I've talked about insurance and I want to give you an idea of what this costs. Because hospital and doctor fees and insurance coverage all vary, it's only meant to give you a general idea. I'm not sure how useful it would be to name my insurer so I won't, but they're a large provider in Nebraska and other states. I'm also not going to give a line by line accounting of every charge from my two-inch thick stack of insurance paperwork such as all the lab work, consultations and follow-up office visits. I will share what was on my insurer's explanation of benefits statement for each of my surgical procedures. Each of these items reflects the total charges, not the net charges (what was actually paid) or not-covered amounts. They include charges for the hospital, various physicians including my surgeons, radiologists and anesthesiologists, nurse anesthetists and pathology.

My first breast-conserving surgery including the wire localization cost $9,179.79.

The second breast-conserving surgery without the wire localization cost $7,118.51.

The mastectomy with first-stage reconstruction was a whopping $42,357.70. While I said I wouldn't itemize these items, one that stands out is the AlloDerm, which accounted for $22,291. When I mentioned that to Robyn on a follow-up visit to Dr. Thompson, she said, "That's why I told him not to drop it on his way downstairs."

The second-stage reconstruction and augmentation surgery cost $20,523.64.

The nipple reconstruction using local anesthetic was a bargain at $3,246.35.

The tattooing cost $175 for each procedure for a total of $350.

This is not comprehensive for the reasons I mentioned, but I came up with a grand total of $82,775.99 (not counting the $4,000 MRI). I've joked that I should take out extra insurance on my chest since it's so valuable now.

The insurance experience brought about another random act of kindness. I was lucky that everything went smoothly on the insurance front with the exception of one entity (not one of my doctors) that was late sending charges. I ended up getting a notice from the insurer that I was responsible so I ended up logging some phone time with both the insurer and medical office.

While I was on the phone waiting for the insurance rep to look something up, she said, "You sound great. How *are* you?" While I was as baffled as usual by the "You sound great" half of that comment—again, how am I supposed to sound?—I told her I felt pretty good. Then she told me that she had a lot of breast cancer in her family so she started getting mammograms in her 20s. She said they told her she was too young and she said, "I don't care, I'm doing it." Bravo for her.

We wished each other well and she gave me tips on what to say to the medical office. God bless her for that since medical billing is one of life's bigger mysteries as far as I'm concerned, and I did a year-long stint writing technical documentation for medical billing software. I never did catch on. (This is a secret about corporate writers, and probably journalists too—we spend a lot of time writing about things we know absolutely nothing about. We're like perpetual students; we learn enough to explain it and then move on.)

The only thing I recall is that in my screen shots of sample medical bills I plugged in all the characters from the TV series *Northern Exposure*, which was big at the time. Dr. Fleischman was the physician and all the other characters were his patients. I don't know if any clients ever noticed. (When you're writing technical documentation, you'll look for just about any way to amuse yourself.)

I am very thankful I have health insurance and I hope that in whatever final form it takes, healthcare reform helps more women (and men and kids) get it. I also hope they keep the stipulation preventing insurance companies from denying coverage to people with pre-existing conditions.

Chapter 6:

How I Spent My Summer Vacation: Coping and Support

Once you join the pink ribbon tribe, those pesky ribbons seem to be everywhere. (I'm just thankful I wasn't diagnosed in October.) That's partly because we tend to notice things that affect us, making them seem more pervasive than they are. But breast cancer has gained so much awareness that it's become a cottage industry. Everything from water bottles to kitchen shears to vacuum cleaners sports a pink ribbon. Sometimes I think it's reached the point of ridiculousness, but then I remember it's all for a good cause.

Bruce and I both felt hounded by pink ribbons in the days immediately following my diagnosis. Some days it made one or both of us feel trapped, others we just found it funny. The one place we did not expect to encounter breast cancer was watching the HBO *John Adams* miniseries. His daughter had breast cancer—so much for escapism. It was okay until they got to the 18th century mastectomy minus anesthetic. Bruce yelled at me to leave the room. When I came back I asked how it was and he said, "I don't know, my eyes were closed."

If you have a partner, cancer affects both of you. Bruce shouldered a pretty big load throughout this process. He went to at least two dozen appointments with me when I was in hamster-wheel mode and when I wasn't allowed to drive. He managed my surgical drains and cooked and cleaned. I told him one day I couldn't have gone through this without him, and could see he was trying not to say he wouldn't have had to go through it without me. We laughed about that.

In the first week or so after I was diagnosed, Bruce left for work at least a couple of times without remembering to lock the back door or take his phone or wallet, which is not like him at all. He was calm on the surface but had his own undercurrents to deal with.

Bruce also had to get used to watching four different doctors examine his wife's chest. A friend asked him if that was weird and he said, "Only the first time."

One particularly bad day, Audrey gave me a basket full of silly stuff including a red rubber Courage bracelet from a local cancer center. Bruce put that bracelet on and wore it 24/7 until we got the all-clear from Dr. Moshman on July 18.

I'm sure there's some subliminal cancer overcompensation quirk at play here, but after I was first diagnosed I could not seem to stop purchasing underwear. I mean really girly lacy stuff. I was particularly obsessed with bras. Every time I noticed a cute one, I bought it. And then I had to buy whatever went with it. And yes, some of it was even pink. This wasn't like me—I mean, if I was going to go on a shopping binge B.C. (Before Cancer) it would be shoes. A.D. (After Diagnosis) it was bras. Go figure.

It may have been a subconscious fear of losing my femininity. I wasn't worried that Bruce wouldn't want me anymore. I didn't see a mastectomy in my future at the time. But I didn't question my impulse; I just started stockpiling underwear like squirrels stockpile acorns. Ours is not to question retail therapy.

Luckily, the underwear mania eventually subsided, and I am not feeling any less feminine now that I've gone through the mastectomy and reconstruction. The funny thing is that I have moved on to collecting sports bras. I had to wear them when Dr. Thompson prescribed them to prevent scar tissue, and discovered they're a lot more comfortable than the underwire rigs I used to wear. I've tried wearing an underwire bra since then but I found I can't really stand them anymore, not to mention I no longer need one.

When you get cancer, you're faced with many decisions aside from bras. One of them is deciding whom to tell, and when, and how. Your good friends and immediate family are no-brainers. It's the rest of the world that gets a bit interesting. It's not exactly elevator conversation.

"What's new?"

"Oh, just a little bout with breast cancer—you?"

Like everything else, it's best to follow your instincts. If you tend to be private in the rest of your life, you'll probably be private about this as well. That's how it was for me. I know that may sound hypocritical coming from someone who splashed her personal story all over a newspaper, blog and book, but I can explain. (And believe me, I haven't included everything. It's possible to tell your story in this tweeting, Facebooking, blogging world while still keeping aspects of yourself private.)

I think of myself as a writer and you should know something about writers. We're braver at the keyboard. There's something wonderfully intimate about writing. There's also something wonderfully anonymous about it. There's me, writing these words, hoping you're there to read them. But I have no way of knowing you did unless you were to tell me after the fact. And there's you, right now, alone with my words. We're together, but we're not. We're not on the elevator.

Part of the reason I bagged on my trip home for my dad's graveside service and nephews' graduation was that I didn't feel ready to tell all the relatives I'd encounter at our family events, nor did I feel capable of maintaining a poker face. (I'm not sure I can blame cancer for that inability.)

The biggest reason for staying home was so I could figure out a course of action, but postponing telling relatives definitely was part of it. I kept remembering my mom's funeral when some random old woman pestered me about Mom's medical condition to the point where I nearly said, "Gee, I'm so sorry I forgot to bring the X-rays for you." The only thing that stopped me was my wish to not embarrass my dad or brother. I was dreading more of the same on this trip. I could see myself whipping up my shirt and yelling, "Want to see my scar?"

When I mentioned my fears to Dr. Moshman, he got kind of wound up, which is rare for him. He said just because someone wants to know what's going on doesn't mean you have to tell them. And he's right.

When I was diagnosed, I told only a handful of people at work, which is pretty much how I handle everything. I have the special few I want to let in on my life and the rest are "Fine, and you?"

When my essays started appearing in the *World-Herald* I knew it meant I was coming out of the closet to some extent. I got calls, e-mails and face-to-face comments from people at work telling me they liked my stories (and yes, a couple of them told me on the elevator). And it was nice. By the time the stories started appearing, the mastectomy was three months behind me, which helped. It's easier talking about my cancer in the past tense, which is where it belongs.

I mentioned that if you have a partner, both of you are going through this. It's their story too, and they need to be able to share it. I knew Bruce told some people at work and they wished me well and that was fine. Then I went to their annual golf event, which raises funds for Nebraska Make-A-Wish, and I've never had so many people hug me. Luckily they all calmed down by the Christmas party.

Figuring out how and when to tell people and realizing I also had to let Bruce tell people, who would then want to hug me, wasn't quite up there with deciding on a course of treatment. But it certainly was part of the adventure, and just one more thing I hadn't considered.

Speaking of hugs, a friend gave me a healing journal with

advice on every page for topics to write about. I'm a snob about writing and don't feel like I need a paint-by-numbers approach, thank you very much. But I did look at it and one section was on the power of hugs. It actually said you should demand a hug from your doctor. I was completely mystified by that. I come from a long line of prairie stoics and I'm more the handshake type. It never would have occurred to me to ask any of my doctors for a hug. I'd be as likely to ask for their car keys or bank statements.

But the nice thing was I didn't have to ask. The last time I saw Dr. Kingston as a patient he asked if he could hug me, and he hugged me again when I interviewed him to fact-check a couple of items I was writing about. His hugs were beyond welcome, and so was the one from Dr. Soori the day he recommended the mastectomy.

I'm not suggesting that any healthcare professionals reading this take up hugging. As long as you genuinely convey that you see us as people and not some statistic in a chart, we'll be happy. But if you get the urge to offer a hug, by all means do so. Some of your patients may be fluent in hugging and won't wait for you but others may not feel it's appropriate to initiate it. They'll appreciate it just the same.

If hugs are comforting, telling your story can be liberating. It wasn't all that long ago that cancer was something that people did not talk about publicly. Obituaries never included the word "cancer." People died "after long illnesses."

Betty Rollin's *First, You Cry* was a groundbreaking book when it was published in 1976. You didn't have your choice of cancer memoirs like you do today, or blogs where we can share our personal stories. People just didn't talk about it. (And oh, how things have changed in terms of medical treatment. She spent a week in the hospital after her mastectomy. I spent the night. I think I would have gone completely stir crazy after a week.)

Ted Kooser has a great poem in the book *Cottonwood County*, originally published 30 years ago, about Cancer being lonely and latching onto a man from a small town. From that point on, wherever Clarence went, Cancer went with him. No one treated Clarence the same anymore, so he blew his brains out with a gun.

Kooser wrote this poem before the culture changed, before Kooser himself had cancer and was open about it, writing poems and giving interviews. I guess when you think about it, seeing those pink ribbons all over the place isn't so bad after all. It certainly could be worse.

But that "Don't ask, don't tell" mindset can linger. I think that's part of the reason I didn't talk about my adventure with many people until some of it was in the rear-view mirror. You don't want people looking at you funny or treating you differently or like you're some kind of victim. I did occasionally catch both men and women sneaking glances at my chest, but that's human nature and harmless. It reminds me a bit of the pre-gravity years, except in those days it was just men who never seemed to look me in the eye.

Don't forget a very important audience for your story—yourself. It really does help to write it down, whether you show it to anyone else or not. It can help you sort out your thoughts or remember something nice that happened. Trust me, the nice moments outweigh the bad ones by far.

That's how I started out. When it was my turn to get cancer, I didn't immediately think, "I've got cancer! I think I'll write a book!" I didn't even intend to get published in the *World-Herald*. Writing was the farthest thing from my mind.

Practically as soon as I was diagnosed, my friend and colleague Trish told me I should start a blog, and she and Mary urged me to write a book. I said no way. Yet I was composing some pretty detailed e-mails and I found myself listing all of my appointments, because I was fascinated by the sheer volume. I was doing research before I knew I was doing research.

I need to write things down to help make sense of the world, so

I did start keeping a journal. I was planning to make it a scrapbook with random thoughts and poems, photos and get well cards and other bits of flotsam like the banking brochure I scribbled my initial notes on when Dr. Moshman broke the news. I only got about four pages into it before the *World-Herald* essay series came along, out of the blue.

While I was hanging out in one of the doctor's waiting rooms, I saw an essay contest in a magazine seeking submissions about the most important day of your life. I thought, "I can do that." The most important day of my life was the day I decided to save it and remove my breast cancer risk. I didn't win the contest, but I sent the essay to the *World-Herald* as background when I suggested they write a news story about DCIS. Instead, they asked if they could run it and invited me to do a series of essays, which evolved into this book.

My point with all this isn't "Hey, look at me!" It's more, "You never know how things will turn out," or as Mary is fond of saying, "Things happen for a reason." Even when you're handed a WTF experience like cancer, good things can happen if you're open to them. I know it's hip to be cynical about this in some circles, but I'm in the opposite camp. I never expected breast cancer to become a source of inspiration for writing, either poetry or prose. I never expected to gain such a huge respect for and fascination with the art and practice of medicine. But it did and I did, and I'm grateful.

I've talked about how this is your story and to a lesser extent, your partner's. You may find a few peripheral people who want to make your cancer experience all about them. A corollary to that group is the people who think you're now somehow obligated to take up the cause or wave the flag.

My experience is probably typical. Nearly everyone wished me well or offered to help, but I had a couple of Flag Wavers and a couple of All About Me's. I finally had to shut down one Flag Waver who kept telling me I should take part in her event. I kept politely saying no and then she asked how I thought I could write about this event if I never attended. I said because I'm not writing about your event.

The All About Me's tend to say things like "I'm hurt you didn't tell me," or "I wish you would have told me," so "I could do this or say that or blah de blah blah blah." It's all about their emotions and reactions. If there's a "How are you?" in there somewhere it's buried pretty well. With them I found it's best to just say thanks and let it drop.

It's natural for people to want to share their stories. Once you share yours you'll be surprised at how many others you'll hear, and how uplifting it is to hear them, but the All About Me crowd is a bit different. Trust your gut; you'll be able to tell who's genuinely sharing and who's trying to relegate you to a bit part in their movie.

Just remember, this is your story. You have the right to share it or not, with whomever you wish.

We've covered how the cancer checklist includes talking, listening, hugging—who knew? The other thing I learned about cancer is it eats up a ton of your time off. Aside from the dozens of appointments, I missed a solid month of work recovering from my two big surgeries. Goodbye, Napa—hello, Omaha medical centers. The souvenirs are a bit different—instead of logo wine glasses you get a surgical bra and implant I.D. card.

When I realized this was how I would be spending my summer vacation, I decided to treat it like one and take pictures. I wanted pictures of my doctors and the nurses and receptionists I got to know. I photographed Dr. Kingston's receptionist first and sort of ambushed her, but Carol was a great sport. After that, I asked and everyone humored me.

I almost didn't do it because I felt so dorky but I'm really glad I did. It makes me happy to look at their pictures now. It may seem odd to want reminders of an experience that wouldn't typically be viewed as positive, but all it reminds me of is how good they were to Bruce and me and how much I came to like them.

Their personalities really shine through in the pictures. Dr. Kingston with his easy grin, Dr. Soori's kind expression and hint of a smile, Dr. Moshman relaxed and smiling, although I like the one of him taking notes best because that's how I always think of him.

Dr. Thompson wins the patience award for this one because I took pictures of him on three different occasions; first by himself, then one with Robyn and one with Barbara. He looks willing but just a bit wary in the first photo I took, when he was alone. That surprised me a bit since he's a talented photographer—the upstairs hallway at his medical building is lined with his photographs—but he told me he wasn't sure he liked being equated with a summer vacation. I told him I wasn't sure I liked it either.

After Dr. Thompson put up with me taking pictures a second time, the photographer in him came out and he suggested I take a series of "construction" shots. We joked about how they'd make an interesting Christmas card photo and I told him he's probably the only one who'd appreciate getting a card like that.

We were on the same wavelength on that one because Bruce did take a series of shots starting with the first surgery. We weren't sure we'd even want them, but decided we might as well because you can't go back after it's changed. I'm glad we did because the "after" pictures are pretty impressive. I don't look like one of those topless native women in *National Geographic* anymore. I can't say that taking pictures helped in the therapeutic sense but I also can't say that it hurt.

I really wanted a picture of Dr. Thompson with his wife Barbara but I never had my camera when she was there and it bugged me that I didn't have a picture of them together. She is beautiful and elegant bordering on regal in appearance, but very sweet and warm. She's one of the most gracious people I've ever met.

I was finally able to get their picture the last time I saw them as a patient. On that last visit, they reminded me I'd need to come in at one, three and five years to follow up on the implants, and she said, "You won't be able to get rid of us that easily." Nor would I want to.

In addition to my medical team and "construction" shots, I took pictures of the friends and family who helped me through my excellent adventure because I probably wouldn't have taken them otherwise. It's far too easy to take the people you see every day for granted.

I like calling my cancer experience an adventure because it was one. Here's another great G.K. Chesterton quote that sums it up: "An adventure is only an inconvenience rightly considered. An inconvenience is only an adventure wrongly considered." Cancer is a jolt, even when caught early like mine was. But you can focus on that, or on your wonderful medical team and the love of your family and friends.

It really is like a vacation. Say it rains on your Disney World trip. You can dwell on the rain, or on the cool Mickey Mouse ponchos they hand out and the short lines for rides. It's up to you.

I mentioned earlier that I relied on music during this adventure—humor was the other thing I really leaned on. When they wheeled Ronald Reagan into surgery after he was shot, he said, "I hope you're all Republicans." I've never come up with anything that good but I do crack jokes to break the ice or control tension, often my own. Sometimes the only power you have over a situation is to laugh at it.

The first time we met Dr. Soori he asked if I had any children from a previous relationship and I said, "None that I know of." I'm pretty sure I stole that from Ellen DeGeneres. When we met Dr. Thompson and he correctly guessed my cup size I said "Well, I used to be a (*) but now I'm a long." I don't recall attempting any lame jokes when we met Dr. Kingston. The defensive urge must not have kicked in.

Dr. Moshman doesn't count because I've been seeing him forever and I occasionally say things just to be ornery. At one point he mentioned something about the possibility of chemo if they found my lymph nodes were affected. Since the sentinel node biopsy was in conjunction with the mastectomy, I asked him if that meant they'd have to reattach the breast so they could treat it. I think he just shook his head and smiled.

I mentioned that I wore silly socks to my first surgery and a "F*ck Cancer" hat to my second. I figured I had to do something since I didn't have any Reagan-esque lines. For the mastectomy, I just wanted to stay tall in the saddle and that's okay too. You can't force funny.

Bruce was a great source of humor throughout this adventure. Waiting to meet three new cancer-related doctors for the first time would have been a tense and lonely experience if he hadn't been with me. I mentioned how he broke the tension before meeting Drs. Soori and Thompson. The first time we saw Dr. Kingston was my first time putting on one of those lovely paper gowns and Bruce took my picture in it while we were waiting in the exam room. We cracked up about that. Dr. Kingston's exam rooms are very close to the waiting room and I'm sure people wondered what the heck was going on.

My doctors all have a good sense of humor, and all of them are intuitive enough to know when to employ it. When we first met Dr. Soori, he was nothing but soothing. And he needed to be because of that first oncology consult. He helped us get through that difficult decision, but on every visit since then we've laughed about something or other, whether comparing notes on how anesthesia affects us or the time he said he'd send his report to Drs. Kingston, Moshman and Thompson. He repeated the names, commented that his was the only name that didn't match and laughed. I told him he could change it to Sooriman.

Dr. Kingston's humor is Cabernet-dry. When we were trying to figure out the recovery timeline for different activities, Bruce asked, "What about showering?" He said, "In general, I approve of it," and flashed his high-beam grin. Bruce chuckled about that all the way home.

I mentioned Dr. Thompson joking about a reconstruction Christmas card and my Harley tattoo. After I wrote my reconstruction essay for the *World-Herald* and used the bowling ball/bowling pin analogy for my temporarily mismatched breasts, he wrote me a nice note saying that was his favorite visual.

That opened the door for me to tell him the one about the couple on their 50th wedding anniversary. They decided to go to the same inn they went to for their honeymoon, and have breakfast in their room nude like they did all those years ago. The wife said, "I'm getting that same warm feeling I got on our honeymoon." The husband replied, "No wonder—one of your breasts is hanging in your coffee and the other one is in your oatmeal." Dr. Thompson laughed and said there's a lot of truth to that. And he ought to know. He certainly countered the effects of gravity on mine. I can hardly wait for my 50th anniversary.

Dr. Moshman has been putting up with my humor for years, but I did learn the hard way that I can't joke about blood clots around him. Well, I actually joked about it to Bruce so what I really learned was not to tell Bruce anything I don't want Dr. Moshman to know. As I mentioned, the Tamoxifen I'm taking increases the risk for blood clots.

I had a bit of mild muscle tightness in my thigh one morning while we were getting ready for work and said, "Gee, I hope it's not a blood clot." (I said I joked about it; I didn't say it was funny.) Later that day I was picking blackberries out in the back yard and Dr. Moshman called my cell phone. He asked me to come in for lab work to test for blood clots. Bruce had obviously ratted on me.

I wondered why the lab technician said, "I hope you brought

plenty of blood with you today," until she pulled out 10 vials. I must have had every clotting test known to mankind. The good news is I have none of the markers they were looking for. The bad news is I think my husband and doctor are colluding against me.

I really can't say enough about how much all four of my doctors helped me through this adventure, and I know how blessed I was to have them. I also know I'm lucky to live in a fairly large city with a reputable medical community. If you live in a smaller town, you may not have the luxury of shopping around until you find someone you like. But I really believe that no matter where they practice, doctors are in medicine because they want to help people. You may have to work a little harder to communicate if your doctor's style doesn't mesh with yours, but it's worth it. *You're* worth it. It's like any other relationship—communicating can be hard work.

And yes, it's a bit more complicated in that doctors are authority figures. I know some very intelligent, educated women who are afraid to speak up when they're in a doctor's office. I'm not sure how we get over that other than to just keep trying and keep talking. The more you do it, the more comfortable you'll become.

I've been reading a lot lately about doctor-patient communication and am hoping that my doctors serve as models. I mentioned before how well they were all able to pick up where we left off during our office visits, in spite of the fact I'm far from their only patient. I'm nothing short of amazed at how well each one of them was able to focus on me once he walked through that door.

We owe it to them, and to ourselves, to be in the moment with them. That means turning off our cell phones and giving them our full attention. It means asking questions and being honest, however, that does not give us license to chew on them or their staff. I said earlier that one day I clammed up after Dr. Moshman said some things I didn't like. I owed it to him to let him know what I was thinking, but I think in hindsight it was probably just as well I didn't. My mood was verging on dangerous that day. I was really afraid if I opened my mouth nothing civil would come out, and he doesn't deserve that. No one does.

I'm lucky because my truly bad days were few and far between, and I'm beyond lucky to have a good outcome. But even at stage 0, cancer is a wake-up call and makes you realize what's important. Reconnecting with friends and family is a more obvious example, but old loves like art and literature may reappear in your life as well.

In my case, I started writing poetry again and it was like reuniting with an old friend. And I was—I was reconnecting with a part of myself that I thought had vanished for good. I hadn't written or published anything in close to 20 years and really believed that part of my life was over. I'm very grateful to have it back.

A few poems were inspired by my excellent medical adventure but most were not. I've sent some of them out to different venues that publish poetry and a handful have been picked up. Many more have been rejected. I just have to keep working and trying to get better. Whether I find homes for more of them or not, I'm having a great time.

As a solitary keyboard jockey, one thing I did not do was join any support groups. If you're social and enjoy groups in other areas of your life, you may enjoy it here as well. Audrey went through A Time to Heal, a 12-week rehabilitative program developed in Omaha to help women with the physical, emotional and spiritual aspects of recovering from breast cancer. (It's since been expanded to women and men with any type of cancer.) She really liked it.

When you join the pink ribbon tribe, a host of special events are geared to you, the Susan G. Komen Race For The Cure being the big one in many communities. I finally went in 2009. I didn't develop a burning urge to take up the cause; my primary reason was to support Audrey, who walks every year, for being such a good friend and mentor. What kept me from it before I was diagnosed was my natural tendency toward laziness. Audrey's group meets at our office at 7 a.m. on the mornings when the walk takes place. It's always on a Sunday and I'm extremely selfish about my Sundays.

The walk was definitely a happening. It's impressive to see so many people gather in one place, and it's a hoot to see the fun people have with it, like the group of women in pink hula skirts. It's kind of humbling to come around a corner and see a cheer squad jumping around and shaking their pom-poms and realize it's for you. And it's completely sobering to see people wearing In Memoriam shirts. I had to work pretty hard to get a grip on myself after following a group of those shirts for a couple of blocks.

I have mixed feelings about all these events. I'm not convinced that breast cancer merits any more attention than lung cancer or the colon cancer that killed my mom. But if all this hoopla helps find a cure, then I'm all for it. And as I mentioned earlier, there's something so deeply personal about breasts. They represent femininity, food, sex and life. It doesn't get more primal than that.

After the walk Bruce and I went shopping at Nebraska Furniture Mart, which is to furniture what Borsheims is to jewelry. It's the place to go in Omaha whether you need a bedroom set or big-screen TV. I had a couple of encounters there that summed up my ambivalence about these things.

We were in the kitchen appliances aisle when we passed a young woman in her white walk T-shirt. She saw me in my pink survivor's shirt and smiled at me. As we were leaving, we passed a young couple in their walk T-shirts pushing a Buick-sized stroller. There was something a bit smug about them; they reminded me of Chevy Chase's next-door neighbors in *Christmas Vacation*. And sure enough, as soon as the guy saw me, he looked away. I know that lack of eye contact is typical when some young people catch sight of older people. As an over-50 woman, I've gotten used to becoming invisible at certain retail outlets. But I can't help feeling they were more interested in being trendy than in being reminded of why they were sporting these T-shirts.

Other big events in Omaha in October 2009 were a university-sponsored luncheon featuring Barbara Delinksy, a survivor and author of the book *Uplift*, and an annual brunch sponsored by a group of doctors and survivors, including Dr. Soori's group. Both were great events but again, I don't know that I want to make it a habit.

I went to both thanks to my friend and hairdresser Barb. She found out in the space of a couple of months that seven of her friends or clients had developed breast cancer, including me. She has developed a real passion for women's health issues, particularly the use of carcinogens in beauty projects.

The thing that struck me most about the luncheon was the beautiful young woman I got to sit next to. She's a social worker at a cancer center, and she's battling stage 3 breast cancer. She has a great hearty laugh and eyes the color of an October sky. I couldn't help but feel humble talking to her. I've had a few other moments like that, when I felt a bit sheepish even thinking of myself as a survivor. When you're battling stage 3 or stage 4 cancer, you know you're in a fight for your life. Since mine was stage 0, I wasn't sure I was entitled to call myself a survivor. I had to remind myself no one is grading on the curve here. And after five surgeries for some very stubborn DCIS I figure I've earned my survivor status.

The thing that stood out most about the brunch, aside from Sylvia McNair's amazing performance (she's also a breast cancer survivor) was the roll call. They started out with survivors of 30 years or more, and made their way through 20, 15, 10, 5 and 1, and then they asked the newly diagnosed to stand and be recognized. A woman at the table next to ours stood up and just dissolved in tears. Barb's friend Kay went over and put her arms around her. I'm not sure there was a dry eye in the ballroom at that point. I know mine weren't. I admired the newbie for her guts. I would have been way too scared to show up at such an event when I first got the news. I hope it helped her; I can't help but think it did.

There's no question breast cancer has become a big deal and it's even generated some pink ribbon backlash, most recently with Barbara Ehrenreich's book *Smile or Die: How Positive Thinking Fooled America And The World*. It was triggered by her experience with breast cancer and the cultural pressure she felt to be cheerful. My take on it is no one should tell us how to feel about our diagnosis. That's kind of like telling someone she should be six feet tall or have brown eyes.

We need to be who we are, handle cancer in whatever way we see fit, and above all respect each other's choices. Cry or laugh, joke or dance, raise money or don't, wear a pink ribbon or not, and choose the doctors and treatment options you're most comfortable with. Shout it from the rooftops or move on and don't look back. The point is to find your own path to peace. As I said when I was discussing the decision roller coaster, once I was able to come to terms with my decision, I was able to find a measure of peace that has not left me.

I realized just how much peace I found when we went out with our friends Janie and Gordon on New Year's Eve, about a month after my second-stage reconstruction and augmentation. While we were having dinner Gordon asked me how I was. I said I was fine, and noticed from the way he was looking at me that he thought I gave a kneejerk answer. Which was not my intention—I just forgot I had any reason not to be fine, and told him so. It was a perfect way to start a new year.

Chapter 7:

What You Need to Know: Interview With My Team

This chapter is my "dream team's" turn to speak. My general surgeon, Tim Kingston; my family doctor, Gordon Moshman; my oncologist, Gamini Soori; and my plastic surgeon, Chester Thompson, answer questions women are likely to ask, sometimes using my case as an example.

About DCIS

Q: What's the most important thing for women diagnosed with DCIS to know?

Dr. Kingston: The main thing is how curable this is and how important early detection is. Mammogram technology has improved tremendously with digital mammograms, and the addition of breast MRIs when the mammogram is not definitive is also helpful. The rate of cure for DCIS is virtually 100 percent. The prognosis has changed dramatically because of early detection.

Dr. Moshman: The most important thing for women with DCIS to know is that this is not invasive, but if not treated properly can progress to invasive in up to 50 percent of cases. It is also unfortunately multicentric, roughly 30 percent of the time. In roughly 40 percent of cases there will be some residual tumor cells remaining at mastectomy, as in your case.

Q: How is DCIS treated?

Dr. Soori: Lumpectomy and radiation or mastectomy with or without reconstruction. You also need Tamoxifen for prevention of occurrence in the other breast.

Dr. Kingston: In general the axillary regional lymph nodes are not evaluated, but there are some exceptions. In your case Dr. Soori recommended it because of the large amount of DCIS and your relatively young age.

Q: How does radiation work and when does it start?

Dr. Moshman: Radiation works by exposing rapidly dividing tumor cells to ionizing radiation, which then destroys their DNA. Optimal timing for radiation is usually three to six weeks after surgery. If a patient would be a candidate for chemotherapy, then radiation, if indicated, would start two to four weeks later depending on the chemotherapeutic agent used.

Dr. Kingston: Radiation therapy is usually started after the patient's range of motion is restored, because the radiation therapist wants a good cushion of wound healing under way before they start the therapy.

Q: Is chemotherapy ever warranted for someone with DCIS?

Dr. Soori: DCIS is by definition a localized form of cancer and is not expected to spread; therefore, it's curable with local treatments such as surgery or radiation therapy.

Dr. Kingston: Chemotherapy is a systemic treatment, meaning it treats the entire body, and DCIS is not a systemic disease. When you treat any kind of cancer, including breast cancer, you're looking at local/regional treatment, which is basically surgery, and systemic treatment if the breast cancer has spread. If the lymph nodes are positive, you have to assume that may have happened.

Q: What are questions you're asked most often by women with this diagnosis?

Dr. Kingston: The most common question is "What's my prognosis?" and most of the time when I see a patient with breast cancer we don't know that yet because we haven't completed surgery and have only done the biopsy. If someone has DCIS, I can tell patients that if no invasive cancer shows up the chance of cure is virtually 100 percent. They also want to know what their diagnosis means to their mother or sister or daughter and what the genetic implications are.

Dr. Soori: Patients are not clear on the difference between DCIS and invasive cancer.

Dr. Moshman: To be honest, when women are first given the diagnosis (and I do not see many people with this), they probably do not make a distinction between invasive and noninvasive cancer and just want it removed. What you say by way of explanation is not processed well. To most people, cancer is cancer.

Q: How does genetic testing work and who should get it?

Dr. Soori: Anyone with a significant family history of cancer or those who are young or have bilateral breast cancer should consider it.

Dr. Moshman: Most breast tumors are not genetic—only 5 to 10 percent are. The test is for BRCA and BRCA 2 genes. Indications include two first-degree relatives (mother or sister) with breast cancer, with at least one diagnosed under 50 years of age; three or more second-degree relatives with breast cancer regardless of age at diagnosis; both breast and ovarian cancer in first- and second-degree relatives; bilateral breast cancer in first- or second-degree relatives; two or more first- or second-degree relatives with ovarian cancer, or breast cancer in a male relative.

The test is not cheap, not foolproof and if positive requires a lot of decisions. I have ordered the test a few times but usually try to develop a family history with a pedigree and have a person see a genetic counselor. Since we do not have health (read: insurance) reform, if the test was positive and the information was known to an insurance company, one might not be able to secure health insurance.

Q: What is the role of clinical trials in cancer and how do they work? Are there any clinical trials for DCIS?

Dr. Soori: Clinical trials are important to learn more about the disease and for treatment of cancer. We are participating in clinical trials for DCIS.

Dr. Moshman: Clinical trials are really what brought us to where we are in cancer treatment. Patients who undergo double blind studies with statistically significant results advance the science, establish new baselines and give us guidelines for treatment. Clinical trials are always ongoing, adding to the data bank of knowledge. Whether we are really anywhere but in the infancy of oncology is hard to say.

In regard to DCIS I am sure there are many ongoing and completed trials. I believe that I cited one trial possibly to you or to one of the physicians connected to your case that radiation was not a substitute for adequate margins and that was why I was pushing for a mastectomy—that came from a controlled but retrospective study. I also know of controlled studies evaluating the addition of Tamoxifen to lumpectomy plus radiation vs. placebo added to lumpectomy plus radiation. This did lower breast cancer events both ipsilaterally (same breast) and contralaterally (opposite breast) when followed for five years.

About Mastectomy and Recovery

Q: Do all patients need physical therapy to restore their range of motion after a mastectomy?

Dr. Kingston: Ninety percent of patients exercise on their own. The other 10 percent use physical therapy, either because they prefer it from the start or don't get results after three weeks of exercising on their own. Some patients request it because they feel like they're going to do better if they've got someone standing over them saying "Here's what you need to do," and there's nothing wrong with that.

Q: I noticed a divot in my armpit after the mastectomy. What caused that?

Dr. Kingston: The breast is teardrop-shaped so you're actually removing breast tissue, not just lymph nodes. The prosthesis should help. What I try to do is make sure the skin in that underarm area is tucked back up the way it normally is after surgery. You don't want that skin hanging down because that's really uncomfortable. The suction from the surgical drains helps the skin heal in that position.

Q: What causes the burning and numbness you get in your armpit and along your arm after surgery?

Dr. Kingston: Skin nerves come out through the chest wall and course through the lymph nodes to go to the underarm area. When you remove lymph nodes, many of those skin nerves are sacrificed. The burning sensation, which can even go down below the elbow, is temporary and due to nerve irritation. The numbness diminishes with time although the nerves don't reappear. There can be some recruitment of other nerves but I think there's also an accommodation factor. Patients get used to it so it doesn't seem to be as severe.

Q: What is lymphedema?

Dr. Soori: Swelling in the arm due to poor fluid drainage from disrupted lymphatics.

Q: Who is most at risk for getting lymphedema?

Dr. Kingston: Patients who have a considerable number of lymph nodes involved, meaning more than three are positive, will be advised to have radiation to the underarm area. The chance of lymphedema is increased if you had radiation to that area.

Dr. Moshman: Sometimes lymphedema doesn't develop for a few years after surgery and radiation. It can be precipitated by low atmospheric pressure such as an airplane flight. Wearing a compression sleeve can be helpful in preventing it.

About Reconstruction

Q: Why was I able to get immediate reconstruction, and who would not be?

Dr. Thompson: Immediate reconstruction is not performed

in patients who have advanced breast cancer and may require immediate post-operative radiation or chemotherapy. Both of these procedures will delay wound healing so reconstruction would be jeopardized.

Q: I've read and heard that you get really good results when the surgeon and plastic surgeon work together for immediate reconstruction—why is that?

Dr. Kingston: There are certain requirements for successful reconstruction and certain requirements for good healing in patients not thinking about reconstruction. With reconstruction, the main thing is making sure there's enough skin to cover the implant or tissue, if tissue replacement is used.

Dr. Thompson: It is important to get surgeons who have worked together for this type of procedure, because it's important that the general surgeon if at all possible leave the pectoralis fascia in place. This is a thin sheet of tough material that covers the pectoralis muscle and prevents it from tearing when we place the prosthesis beneath it. Some surgeons are not very careful about preserving the fascia, thus making the first stage of reconstruction very difficult to achieve.

Q: The two choices in implants are saline and silicone—What are the key differences between them?

Dr. Thompson: Silicone has a much more natural tactile feel and appearance in the reconstructed breast. Because the tissue is quite thin after a mastectomy, a saline implant has small folds due to the fact it cannot be completely expanded, or it becomes too firm. These ridges can be seen through the skin and have an abnormal feel.

Q: How does tissue replacement surgery work and how is that different from using implants? What are the pros and cons of each? Is there more than one kind of tissue replacement surgery?

Dr. Thompson: Sometimes tissue expansion is not possible in a person with an irradiated chest or one with very thin tissues following mastectomy. Tissue replacement can be done in several ways. A patient can have a "tram" flap from the abdomen, which is a large "paddle" of tissue including skin, fat and muscle that is transferred from the abdomen to the mastectomy site. This leaves a football-shaped scar on the reconstructed breast and does not require a prosthesis.

"Free" flaps are performed by a team of surgeons using microscopes to connect vessels. It's very difficult and time-consuming and requires several days in the hospital. Both of these procedures have many more potential complications than tissue expansion.

The (tissue expansion) procedure you had is direct, has few complications and has only one scar on the chest, which is the original mastectomy scar. All procedures are performed through that incision. The prostheses that are available now are very realistic, and one can achieve a very natural appearing breast in a shorter period of time with far fewer complications.

Q: How does the tissue expander work?

Dr. Thompson: The tissue expander is placed beneath the pectoralis major muscle to protect the implant from eroding through the thin tissue remaining after the mammary gland was removed in the mastectomy. One can picture a tissue expander as a deflated balloon, which will be slowly inflated over several months. This stretches the surrounding muscles and skin to allow insertion of a permanent breast implant, much like pregnancy slowly stretches the abdomen.

Q: What is AlloDerm and when is it indicated for use in reconstruction?

Dr. Thompson: AlloDerm is irradiated human tissue used to help enlarge the pocket created in the pectoralis muscle, to give a more natural appearance to the inferior pole of the reconstructed breast and allow better tissue expansion. Since you had a relatively large opposite breast, I used it to enlarge the pocket and support a larger tissue expander.

Q: What are some misunderstandings women have about reconstruction?

Dr. Thompson: Some people believe that the reconstructed breast will appear the same as before the mastectomy. Sometimes it looks even better, but women should be aware that this is not always possible and should understand the limitations. Also, in no other field of surgery is the word "art" more applicable than plastic surgery. Not all surgeons who have passed their boards are artistic or have the dexterity to do these complicated procedures. The patient needs to explore her options with several surgeons or at least be satisfied that referrals are from advisors or friends she can trust.

Q: My mastectomy implant was placed inside a pocket you created in the chest wall but my augmentation implant was not— why the difference? Is it because of the mastectomy?

Dr. Thompson: The mastectomy pocket has only muscle to protect the implant from a very thin layer of skin and subcutaneous fat after the breast gland has been removed. As I mentioned, I used AlloDerm to help enlarge the pocket for a more natural appearance and better tissue expansion.

On your right side you had quite a bit of soft tissue so I didn't need to bury the implant beneath your pectoralis muscle. The submuscular implant is necessary in some cases to help smooth the upper end of the implant. This prevents the "grapefruit" look that is so common on actresses and models.

Q: What is the process used in nipple reconstruction?

Dr. Thompson: The star flap technique is like using the upper half of a five-pointed star with the two lateral flaps wrapped around the central core. The top point is then bent over and attached to lateral flaps, thus creating the nipple. People used to use skin grafts from the labia because of its dark nature but this has been totally replaced by nipple creation and tattooing.

The star flap procedure is usually performed with the base right on the mastectomy scar, as this is where the previous nipple had been located. I always ask women if they would like to partake in locating nipples and most defer to me, however, I think it gives them the chance to feel involved in the final act of reconstruction.

Q: Do most women opt for nipple reconstruction or do they skip that step?

Dr. Thompson: I would say at least half of my patients opt for nipple reconstruction. I try to persuade them to have it performed as I think it helps them feel more normal and lose the stigma of mastectomy.

Q: What do women need to know about having the other breast lifted (mastopexy) and augmented with an implant?

Dr. Thompson: It takes considerable artistic sense and experience for a reconstructive surgeon to visualize how to lift, tighten and augment the "normal" breast to match the reconstructed breast. On the reconstructed breast, the implant elicits a tissue reaction that prevents the implant from dropping. The mastopexy lifts and tightens the other breast to provide better symmetry.

Q: What are some things women want to know/should know about reconstruction that I haven't asked?

Dr. Thompson: Choosing the right reconstructive surgeon should not be taken lightly. It's extremely important to seek out the best in that field, just as it is to find a general surgeon for mastectomy. Patient or doctor referrals are very important and the patient should feel comfortable with the doctor she chooses. Also, the patient and reconstructive surgeon need to coordinate their thoughts about the implant size before final implant placement. Many different implants are now available.

Some people seem put off by the amount of time reconstruction takes—typically six to eight months—but when one considers a lifetime this goes by quickly and will soon be forgotten.

About Communication

Q: It can be hard to communicate well when you've been hit with a big diagnosis like cancer. Got any tips for us on how to communicate effectively with you? What are some things you've learned about communicating with us?

Dr. Soori: We need to communicate with you in stages—first broad generalities, then more specifics. We need to understand each patient's ability to comprehend issues and information. We also need to repeat it because they won't understand all they hear and will remember even less. For patients, it's good to write down your specific questions.

Dr. Moshman: Communication is difficult. The patient has to be ready to listen, there needs to be the right atmosphere and there needs to be a mutual respect and understanding. The word "doctor" means to teach in Greek and some of what we do is teaching and advising. Given the time restraints, distractions, beepers, cell phones, it can be difficult. Sometimes patients don't hear anything you said other than using big words, and get angry. Sometimes I will call them up as I did you just to make sure they understand and to see if they now have any questions, and I do this after office hours when one can talk without expected interruptions.

Dr. Thompson: I know this is a very emotional time for women and many times they arrive with no previous knowledge of reconstruction. I think this is fine, as some of them are still in a state of shock. The reconstructive surgeon should spend whatever time it takes to answer their questions and to reassure them that a great deal can be achieved toward developing a "normal" looking breast.

Q: Does being able to research our conditions on the Internet make your job easier or more difficult?

Dr. Soori: It is good to know more about one's cancer and treatments. Because sources of information on the Internet may not be reliable or authoritative, you should check with your doctors before you make decisions.

Dr. Moshman: The Internet has some reputable sites that educate patients and help them take better care of themselves. It also has some complete trash put out by inexperienced, uninformed users, often with some other agenda. So it can be helpful but also harmful.

Warrior Princess

—for Pam

Those long legs carried her across the Chiefs parking lot,
battle veteran, blond head held high,
rebuilt breasts the prow of a proud ship.
As she passed, men's necks snapped around
like rows of sunflowers following the sun.

Now those legs carry her through the halls of chemo,
bald head and fists high as she stares down the Beast.
She girds herself for the daily bombardment
of pelvis and spine by radiation,
chemo drip in the La-Z-Boy showroom from Hell,
armed only with that spirit blazing like a star.
Slayer of pity, resister of the morphine cloud,
she says she's going to play the hand that's dealt her.
I wouldn't bet against her.

Some Useful Resources

I found the following books and Web sites to be helpful as I was researching my breast cancer.

> *The Breast Cancer Survival Manual, Fourth Edition: A Step-by-Step Guide For The Woman With Newly Diagnosed Breast Cancer* by John Link, M.D. (Owl Books)
> *Dr. Susan Love's Breast Book* by Susan Love, M.D., with Karen Lindsey (Da Capo Press)
> *Nordie's At Noon* by Patti Balwanz, Kim Carlos, Jennifer Johnson and Jana Peters (Da Capo Life Long)
> *First, You Cry* by Betty Rollin (Harper Paperbacks)
> www.mayoclinic.com
> www.webmd.com
> www.breastcancer.org

I've become hooked on these blogs from doctors who are out there in the trenches. I've posted comments on occasion and I would encourage you to do the same. Plus, I just love reading these guys.

> www.distractiblemind.org
> www.33charts.com
> www.mdwhistleblower.blogspot.com

Poetry Web sites that have absolutely nothing to do with cancer (because we all need a break).

> www.rattle.com
> www.poetryfoundation.org
> www.ploughshares.com

While it may be a stretch to call it useful, please feel free to visit my blog at http://secondbasedispatch.com so we can keep the discussion going. I'd love to hear from you. You can also visit my Web site at www.fromzerotomastectomy.com.

Other helpful resources:

Pink-Link (www.pink-link.org) is like Match.com for survivors and caregivers.

PEG'S Group (www.pegsgroup.com) provides resources to survivors in NYC and beyond.

Both CURE and Breast Cancer Wellness offer free print magazine subscriptions to cancer survivors (www. CUREtoday.com and www.breastcancerwellness.org)

CPSIA information can be obtained at www.ICGtesting.com
Printed in the USA
239893LV00001B/308/P